AF327291

THE SYNTHESIS OF SELF

VOLUME 2
IT ALL DEPENDS ON HOW YOU LOOK AT IT
Development of Pathology in the Cohesive Disorders

THE SYNTHESIS OF SELF
Roy M. Mendelsohn, M.D.

THE SYNTHESIS OF SELF

VOLUME 2
IT ALL DEPENDS ON HOW YOU LOOK AT IT
Development of Pathology in the Cohesive Disorders

ROY M. MENDELSOHN, M.D.

PLENUM MEDICAL BOOK COMPANY
NEW YORK AND LONDON

Library of Congress Cataloging in Publication Data

Mendelsohn, Roy M.
  The synthesis of self.

  Contents: v. 1. The I of consciousness—v. 2. It all depends on how you look at it—
v. 3. Believing is seeing—[etc.]
  Includes bibliographies and index.
  1. Self. 2. Psychology, Pathological. 3. Psychotherapy. I. Title. [DNLM: 1. Con-
sciousness. 2. Personality Disorders. 3. Psychoanalytic Theory. 4. Psychoanalytic
Therapy—methods. WM 190 M537s]
RC455.4.S42M46   1987   616.89   87-25798
ISBN 0-306-42711-7 (v. 1)
ISBN 0-306-42712-5 (v. 2)
ISBN 0-306-42713-3 (v. 3)
ISBN 0-306-42714-1 (v. 4)

© 1987 Plenum Publishing Corporation
233 Spring Street, New York, N.Y. 10013

Plenum Medical Book Company is an imprint of Plenum Publishing Corporation

Printed in the United States of America

To my teachers:

my family who taught me to love,
Missy who taught me about autonomy,
Rebel who taught me about life,
and my patients who taught me what to write

Overview of *The Synthesis of Self*

This series consists of four volumes. Volume 1 addresses healthy development, moving from the earliest, most primitive stages to the most advanced stages, culminating in a picture of the genital character. The therapeutic progress of an autistic child is presented to illustrate the various developmental steps negotiated during the course of his treatment, supplemented by clinical material from others demonstrating similar points.

Volumes 2 and 3 address the pathological consequences of an inability to negotiate specific developmental tasks, moving from those with the most advanced psychic organization to those with the most primitive, culminating in a description of the autistic disorders. There was a natural division into two volumes owing to the crucial significance of cohesiveness for determining the conditions necessary to facilitate constructive growth. Some clinical material from Volume 1 is used to bring out the full picture of the pathology, which had only been alluded to in the earlier volume because of its focus on healthy processes.

Volume 4 addresses the basic principles of psychoanalytic treatment and their applicability across the broad spectrum of pathology, moving from the most primitive autistic disorders to the most advanced hysterical disturbances, to explicate the essence of the principles and their evolution into a classical psychoanalytic posture. Some clinical material from Volumes 1–3 is included to demonstrate the effects of the therapeutic relationship—when guided by the basic psychoanalytic principles in accordance with their essential nature—on both healthy and pathological processes.

The use of several patients' psychic productions throughout the series of four volumes illuminates the interweaving of healthy and pathological forces operative in a given individual, highlights their significance in guiding a therapist toward conducting a growth-promoting therapeutic relationship, and provides a thread of continuity connecting health, pathology, and treatment.

Roy M. Mendelsohn, M.D.

St. Louis

Preface

The oedipal situation involves much more than an instinctual attitude toward a prohibited object giving expression to unconscious wishes. It introduces a whole new way of perceiving the internal and external world and an entirely different orientation to the myriad of life's experiences. A great deal of structural development, requiring the negotiation of a sequence of early developmental tasks, has to have taken place before it is possible to encompass the complex demands of an oedipal attitude. When these early steps are not negotiated, although genital instinctual impulses may be manifested, the structural alignments necessary to enter into an oedipal position cannot be effected and the intrapsychic conflicts it engenders are not encountered. The thrust of early development has made it essential for a narcissistic perspective to be adopted toward all stimuli and all relationships in order to enable continuing self-expansion. All attachments must of necessity be based upon the narcissistic supplies they contain, which ultimately lead to increasing levels of independence, self-differentiation, and individuation. It is precisely when the component instincts are consolidated into a genital drive that a narcissistic orientation can no longer incorporate the representation of experiences needed for the full realization of self-potentials. Were stimuli to only possess significance in regard to their narcissistically enhancing attributes, the resulting dependence upon the external world would run counter to the thrust for independence and autonomy. The transition from narcissism to object relatedness is equally a transition from needing to be loved by an object to developing the capacity to be enhanced by loving an object. This places separateness and autonomy on a more solid and independent basis, allowing greater freedom in object choice and a more complete realization of dormant mental functions. The oedipal situation presents a potential pathway for fulfilling this developmental task by organizing a new level of psychic structuralization that enables the unseen dimensions of experience to be represented, adding richness to love relationships and broadening the autonomous functions of the ego. The hysteric and obsessive have been able to manage the transition to object relatedness with an inordinate degree of conflict, leaving infantile attachments that if unchanged will interfere with continuing progression. The phobic remains fixated in the transitional phase, with the oedipal situation representing an overwhelming demand.

This volume presents an in-depth study of psychological disturbances in the cohesive personality, signifying that the self- and object systems of representation are structurally united and differentiated, continuity of experience is established, and repression proper functions as the major ego defense. The effects of a lack of synchrony in stage and phase specificity during the pregenital period are explored, and the pathology manifested with the formation and lack of resolution of an oedipal conflict is explicated. The relationship of character defenses to character pathology in the obsessive and hysteric is defined, and the significance of symptom formation illuminated. Discussion of the phobic disorders is particularly relevant because it clarifies an area clouded with uncertainty. Through an exposition of the nature of the unstable structures maintaining cohesiveness, the shifting positions, from exhibiting threats to self integrity to representing instinctual dangers are explained, reflecting the difficulty in negotiating the transition from narcissism to object relatedness. The role of the fixation points in creating distortions when defensively maintained is delineated, highlighting the foundation on which pregenitally determined character attitudes and defenses against the transference are constructed. The pathological consequences of an inordinately conflicted oedipal situation are revealed in the overdeveloped incestuous fantasies expressive of defense transferences, the dangers associated with primal scene fantasies expressive of the transference, and the immature level of superego consolidation expressed through harsh prohibitions and a polarization of functions. The differences between hysteric and obsessive configurations are portrayed, and the relationship of character pathology to symptom formation is described. The phobic disorders are referred to as narcissistically determined and object related; they are the equivalent of cohesive, narcissistic personality disorders and exist on a fluctuating continuum of pathology. The underlying basis for the phobic attitude toward the influences of a bad object and toward instinctual overstimulation is presented. The hysteric, obsessive, and phobic disorders have all advanced sufficiently to move toward an object-related orientation, but this orientation has been unsuccessful to a greater or lesser degree in mastering its demands.

Roy M. Mendelsohn, M.D.
St. Louis

Contents

Contents of Other Volumes

Volume 3
Believing Is Seeing: Pathology of
Development in the Noncohesive Disorders

Volume 4
The Principles That Guide the Ideal Therapist

Introduction

Psychological growth is an amalgam of healthy and pathological forces. The various manifestations of pathology occur on a background of developmental experiences, and it is important in formulating the sequential evolution of a given psychic event to discriminate between healthy and distorted lines of development. There are crucial periods when an inability to negotiate or master a particular developmental phase, stage, or task leads to similarities in the psychological processes utilized in adaptive functions and in the way stimuli are registered. Although they are unique in each individual, the similarities reflect the psychological foundation upon which diagnostic categories are constructed. Pathological entities can be formulated as the product of difficulty in mastering developmental tasks at crucial phases, and they emerge in a hierarchy that expresses an advance in the stages of development. This presentation will focus attention upon those tasks that have not been adequately mastered after the point in development when cohesiveness has been established.

Progressive steps in development are affected by the manner in which earlier steps have been negotiated, and the point at which pathological distortions evolve leaves a unique imprint that continues to exert an influence. In the cohesive disorders, the debilitating and distorting effects of pathology are not manifested until after the process of separation–individuation has been successfully negotiated, although the manner in which it takes place plays a decisive role in determining the particular constellations of pathology that are organized. In this presentation, I will define the significance of cohesiveness, the manner in which it is formed, and its effect upon mastering the developmental tasks that are negotiated after it has been attained.

The mental representational world is comprised of two realms of experience that reflect the activity of perceptual processes in registering stimuli and evoking the representational and organizational functions of the ego. Body ego experiences are at the foundation of a self-system of representations, and their object-impression counterparts are at the foundation of an object system of representations. Initially, they are fused and inadequately distinguished, gradually coalesce into separate and distinct entities, and finally are united and differentiated from each other. The varied aspects of self-experience and the differing impressions of an object's influence are elaborated into fantasies, which function as the unifying and differentiating linkages between the two realms of mental experiences. Cohesiveness is established with the structuralization of these linkages during the processes of separation and individuation.

The title of this volume, *It All Depends on How You Look at It*, expresses the concept that a given stimulus can be perceived in different ways depending upon the attitude of the observer. It also embodies the idea that a given stimulus can be perceived in differing ways simultaneously. The capacity to perceive differing stimuli, and simultaneously the same stimulus in differing ways, requires an interrelationship to exist between perceptual functions and mental representations that are formed by them. Each has an influence upon the other, and the manner in which a stimulus is perceived is determined by the degree of freedom from the effects of memory traces. The evolution of a unified and differentiated system of self- and object representations is interwoven with the delineation of a continuum of perceptual functions, possessing differing qualities, which define the systems of conscious, preconscious, and unconscious mental activities. This is a necessary precondition for this complex act of perception to be accomplished. When cohesiveness has not been established, everything does not depend upon how you look at it. Continuity of experience is not present within the personality, the primitive level at which the representations of the self and object are organized disrupts the function of perception, and everything depends upon being able to perceive. The ability to simultaneously perceive differing aspects of a stimulus, and to perceive a stimulus in differing ways, is either absent or severely impaired.

Each individual has a unique and idiosyncratic personality makeup, but there are similarities in psychological functioning that allow diagnostic categories to be formulated. These diagnostic categories will be described on a developmental hierarchy, extending from the most advanced to the most primitive in organization.

The Genital Character

The genital character represents the most advanced level of psychic organization and is the healthy outcome of stage and phase specificity in the sequences of development. A genital character can be defined by the manner in which the major experiences of work, play, and love are included in an individual's life. Each of these experiences requires the smooth and harmonious functioning of all psychic processes and adaptational mechanisms, to be fully realized. A hallmark of the genital character is the selection of love relationships, play activities, and work situations that express all dimensions of the personality, are balanced in their proportions, and enhance a continuing process of self-expansion.

Work performances and achievements are not experienced as proof of strength or power but provide narcissistic gratification. These narcissistic elements are not compensatory in nature and include involvement with an object. Superego responses are not overly prohibitive but are regulatory and guiding. The ego ideal, based upon discriminating selective identifications, is guided by the participation of a conflict-free sphere of functioning. The realizable potentials of the self are in close approximation to the fantasy elaborations utilized in establishing selective identifications. Aggression is differentiating, freely expressed through self-assertiveness, and there is ample energy for affective experiences and realistic actions in the external world. Actions and experiences are intense and spontaneous. There is a capability for adaptive, defensive responses with flexibility and control. The genital character can be joyful but also angry, and experiences of loss are reacted to with depression without being enveloped by it. There is an openness to the external world that can be as intense in one situation, as the ability to shut off the impact of the external world is in another. The expression of courage is not a compensatory act but is in the service of attaining a goal.

Instinctual activity is well regulated, granted sublimatory expression through a structured integrated pathway, and gentle restraint is available when necessary. Varying levels of neutralized instinctual energy expressed through the pregenital component instincts are allowed gratification under selected conditions. The genital character can be childlike without being infantile, seriousness is natural, and there is a capacity for intense love and also for intense hatred. The ego is operative upon a solid foundation, and relationships with the external world are based upon a realistic orientation guided by the participation of a conflict-free sphere of functions.

Love relationships are genitally determined, relatively free of ambivalence, and object-seeking behavior is no longer directed by incestuous and rivalrous strivings. Genital interest is in new heterosexual objects, which are freed of the influence of infantile attachments. The oedipal conflict has served its organizing function in enabling the shift from narcissism to object relatedness, and the importance of being loved by the object has changed to being able to love the object. Pregenital instinctual activities are sublimated and gratified in the act of forepleasure. The sexual act itself offers the greatest pleasure and is the most important sexual goal. In the genital sexual act with a loved partner, the ego is capable of being reduced to the function of perception. The individual can be engulfed by pleasure without the presence of anxiety or the need for excessive defense.

Hysteria

Throughout the literature, there has been much discussion and confusion concerning the diagnosis of hysteria. Freud (1901–1905/1953) originally stressed the repression of infantile sexual wishes that was involved in hysterical symptoms and the multi-determined nature of those wishes. This led to numerous psychoanalytic formulations of hysterical symptoms as infantile sexual strivings that were unable to attain sublimatory expression due to the oedipal fear of punishment or disapproval from the parent of the same sex. The resulting conflict was portrayed as leading to a regression that produced the symptoms. A classic example was of *globus hystericus,* in which sexual excitement was displaced from the genitals and vomiting reflected a concern over oral impregnation. Fenichel (1945) described the oedipal complex as the nuclear complex in all neuroses and particularly emphasized its validity in hysteria. He stressed the fixation to the phallic phase of psychosexual development. However, numerous authors began to direct attention to the preoedipal conflicts that were manifested in hysteria. At first, these were primarily thought of as regressions from the oedipal struggle, rather than as fixations at earlier developmental levels. Many analysts questioned the ease of treatability and the exclusively oedipal conceptualization of causative factors.

As early as the 1930s, Reich (1933) pointed out the pregenital strivings that were a part of the hysterics character makeup. Questions, confusion, and uncertainty arose concerning the diagnosis and underlying dynamics of what had been described as hysterical phenomena. Marmor (1953) emphasized the oral mechanisms and orally influenced symptoms that were always conspicuous and decribed the sexuality of the hysteric as a sham expressing a pregenital oral rather than a genital wish. He still considered the oedipal conflict to be predominant but thought these early oral fixations gave it a pregenital cast. In recent years, the pregenital components of hysterical symptoms were commented on more frequently in conjunction with the primitive types of object relations seen in periods of regression. The emerging picture was of a spectrum of disturbances, all exhibiting hysterical symptoms, which appeared to encompass a wide variety of pathological states. The controversy directed attention to a developmental view of hysterical phenomena. A greater degree of discrimination became possible as the overall functioning of the ego was focused upon. The hysteric's characteristic way of conceptualizing inner experience, overemphasis upon dramatic acts, and behavioral patterns of excitability and emotional unstability were particularly noted. Analytic investigations amplified these behavioral descriptions and identified the disordered perceptual, cognitive, and verbal communication patterns. This seemed to offer a guideline for formulating more decisive explanations as to the underlying dynamics of this disorder.

Horowitz (1977) categorized the hysterics functioning into long-term, medium-term, and short-term patterns. *Long-term patterns* referred to the repetitive relationships that were motivated by infantile attachments. *Medium-term patterns* referred to attention-seeking behavior, suggestibility, and what has been variously described as provocativeness or seductiveness. Characteristically, the hysteric has an absence of any recognition of intent. *Short-term patterns* referred to a communicative style in which the use of language is unclear and imagery is emphasized. Other analytic authors defined the defensive organization of the hysteric, stressing the effects of denial and repression upon actions, thoughts, and ways of processing and organizing information. Shapiro (1965) described the global perceptual manner of the hysteric and the impressionistic grouping of constructs and shallow repertoire of memories.

Sperling's (1973) depiction of the pregenital aspects in hysteria were the most extreme. She accentuated the primitive and destructive meaning of hysterical symptoms and portrayed the quality of the hysteric's object relationships as a special form of symbiotic interaction. The overt expression of aggression and self-assertion was not permitted, and a premium was placed on submission and dependence. This was hypothesized as the developmental underpinning for the formation of an hysterical character. Conversion symptoms were then only understandable in the context of the early mother–child relationship. In Sperling's view, conversion was only possible when there was a regression to pregenital symbiotic phases of development. This helped to clarify the confusion that arose when conversion symptoms were equated with the concept of hysteria.

Hysteria was better understood by defining the overall psychic organization of the personality. It then became apparent that hysterical symptoms could occur in a wide variety of personalities. The question emerged as to how a similar symptom picture could be manifested, when the underlying structures were so different. Much effort was expended in attempting to explain this phenomenum. Many indicated that a diagnosis of hysteria on the basis of symptoms, in such a disparate variety of personalities, was probably inaccurate. Others differentiated between a "good genital hysteric" and a "bad oral hysteric." The differences reflected the degree of ego maturation, and pointed to the need for a developmental understanding of the mental structures at the foundation of an individual's character. Rangell (1959) felt that the mechanism of conversion was employed to express forbidden wishes and was capable of encompassing the entire gamut of psychopathological entities. The classical theory of hysteria, as a genital libidinal fixation manifesting incestuous strivings, was gradually widened to include the pregenital elements. Greater emphasis was placed upon the oral fixations, and a relationship was noted with addictions, depressions, and even schizophrenia.

The varied pathological configurations that had been diagnosed as hysteria, based only upon the symptom, were predominantly manifesting distortions in the representation of self-experience. When this observation is placed in the context of a develomental perspective upon mental structure formation, it is possible to discern the components of what is specifically hysteric in nature. The significance of hysterical symptoms and hysterical character pathology can then be determined because a particular symptom has to be considered within the framework of the underlying character structure. Continued refinement in clinical descriptions of patients and a deeper understanding of the concept of character have made these distinctions possible. The hysteric thinks and communicates with imagery, whereas ideas, concepts, and facts are not easily available. There is a relative absence of cognition and active concentration, and a susceptibility to the transient effects of subjective inner experience. Extreme emotionality is a reflection of this overdetermined focus upon the representations of self-experience. The subjective world is vividly present, with only limited access to intellectual processes that would provide a conceptual grasp of reactions and behavior.

Zetzel (1968), in attempting to reconcile the wide variation in character and personality structure, divided hysteria into subtypes. A "good" hysteric was defined as having genital and oedipal conflicts and mature personality structures. These patients did well in psychoanalytic treatment. A "bad" hysteric was defined as having preoedipal conflicts and defects in personality structure. These patients did poorly in psychoanalytic treatment. Lazare (1971) elaborated upon the developmental, characterological, and behavioral aspects of this hysterical continuum. "Good" hysterics had adequate early mothering, their symptoms were isolated and ego alien, the sexual difficulties were genital and secondary to inhibitions, and behavior was well modulated. "Bad" hysterics had inadequate mothering during early developmental periods, sexuality was perverse, and behavior was blatant and based upon a pervasive personality disorder. Blocker and Tupin (1977) understood the symptom as an expression of the functioning or malfunctioning of the underlying character and in this way explained how symptoms identified with hysteria can be seen in a variety of character structures. The equation of hysteria with hysterical symptoms had contributed much to the confusion in understanding the variability in the conflicting theoretical hypotheses as to its causation. A tendency has remained to consider them as varied expressions of the same underlying disorder in personality or character formation, in spite of the increasing evidence that the opposite ends of the continuum are a product of differing disorders. The confusion tends to be perpetuated by the manner in which the orality of the hysteric is understood. When this oral influence is seen as the consequence of libidinal overstimulation during the early phases of development, coloring predominantly phallic and genital conflicts, the symptoms and character structure that result are of a "good" hysteric. When the orality is seen as the consequence of deprivation during the oral period, creating severe impairments in ego functioning, the symptoms and character structure that result are of a "bad" hysteric.

Easser and Lesser (1965), in responding to this difficulty, described the hysterical personality as differing in regard to object relations, mechanisms of defense, levels of fixation, and ego integration. They used the term *hysteroid* to differentiate the more infantile, borderline, or psychotic personality. Abse (1974) used the term *hysteriform borderline personality* to distinguish those individuals with pronounced oral character traits and a severe narcissistic ego disorder. Berger (1971) also divided hysteria into two subtypes: a genital oedipal and an oral preoedipal. However, he added that if the oral hysterics were as different from the true hysterics as they appeared to be, they should not be subsumed under the same label. Kernberg (1976) indicated that the hysteric individual has healthy, integrated, internalized object relations and an ability to form good interpersonal relationships. He contrasted this with what he called the fluid hysteric, who has the psychic organization of a borderline or narcissistic character disorder.

It is clear that conversion symptoms occur across a wide variety of psychopathological entities. This ranges from the object-related, genitally organized hysteric through those individuals with a narcissistic orientation and extends to the borderline personality and even the catatonic schizophrenias. The one aspect clearly identifiable as common to all is the phenomenum of the body's processes manifesting the effects of a psychic disturbance. This common factor can provide a foundation for a clearer understanding of the similarities and differences between hysteria and the other disorders confused with it. When conversion symptoms are in evidence, it is the structural organization of the personality that is the determining factor as to diagnosis.

Dissociative reactions have also commonly been associated with the diagnosis of hysteria and have been identified as occurring across the same wide spectrum of pathology. However, the only aspect of similarity is the use of a process that excludes competing and contradicting tendencies. Dissociative reactions can only be found in more primitively organized personalities because the process of splitting is required as a major ego defense. Hysteria is an object-related, neurotic disorder in which repression proper is the major defense of the ego. Cameron (1963) discussed this tendency to link dissociative reactions with hysteria. He pointed out that with conversions, most of the personality is left intact, whereas dissociations encompass large segments of reality and are much closer to the psychoses.

The seeds of pathology are formed during the course of development, and psychoanalytic investigators have offered a wealth of information concerning the evolution of the component instincts and their consolidation into a genital drive, the developmental lines of ego functions, and the manner in which an infantile neurosis manifests its effects in childhood. The concept of fixation points has been an integral facet of this developmental perspective. I have defined *fixation points* from a perceptual point of view and formulated their interrelationsihp with character formation. This has particular relevance for determining the structural composition of the cohesive disorders, of which the hysterias are the most advanced.

In healthy development, the fixation points are formed sequentially in a phase- and stage-specific manner. At the end of the oral period, the recognition of a separate good object's influence forms a fixation point on the projective arm of perception, which is stabilized in the anal period by an awareness of the good object's bad qualities. The effect is to anchor object constancy, provide the stability necessary for the grandiose self and ego ideal to be structured, and to maintain differentiation and support projective processes. A fixation point on the introjective arm of perception is formed during the phallic period by an awareness of the good self's bad instinctual qualities. The effect is to provide the stability necessary for castration anxiety to consolidate as a signaling, regulatory structure, and for the oedipal conflict to exert its organizing function. This orderly, phase-specific sequence enables the genital fantasies of the oedipal conflict to structuralize a pathway of instinctual integration and a new boundary for the unconscious system. The consequence is in the ability to register and represent the unseen dimension on the continuum of biophysiological demand and the independent qualities of an object. With the resolution of the oedipal conflict, through selective identifications, the shift from narcissism to object relatedness is fully negotiated. The superego emerges as an independently functioning regulatory and guiding agency, acting in harmony with the interests of the ego. Changes can then take place in the fixation points, which free them from the influences of infantile experience. The fixation point on the projective arm of perception is increasingly depersonified, loosening the attachment to infantile objects. The fixation point on the introjective arm of perception, which has to be transiently maintained for stability during the period of oedipal organization, is integrated, attains secondary autonomy, and is relinquished. The introjective arm of perception is then open to register new object-related experiences without the distorting effect of memory.

Libidinal overstimulation during the earliest phases of the hysteric's development has resulted in a delay in the recognition of a separate good object's influence. That delay has an effect upon the nature of the good object's bad qualities, and the initial fixation point established on the projective arm of perception is based upon a phallically determined attachment. It also affects the structural composition of the grandiose self and ego ideal and delays the formation of a fixation point on the introjective arm of perception until late in the phallic period at the point of a genital consolidation. The emphasis upon orality is reflected in the mental representations that occupy the id of the dynamic unconscious, which tends to give an oral cast to all instinctual experience. Phallic instinctual activity is accentuated and poorly regulated. Castration anxiety consolidates as an unduly prohibitive structure, and the oedipal fantasies elaborated with a genital consolidation are inordinately conflicted. The degre of oedipal conflict resolution is either limited or absent, and the fixation point on the introjective arm of perception must be defensively maintained. There may be some limited oedipal conflict resolution, resulting in a partial integration of the fixation point on the introjective arm of perception. However, this takes place without the regulation of an effectively functioning superego. New object-related experiences are registered that serve as a source of overstimulation, and the compromises of hysterical symptoms are formed in place of processes of sublimation. Early developmental events have led to a preponderance in the representation of orally influenced, phallically determined body ego experiences, which are at the foundation of conversion symptoms. The individual with hysterical symptoms has attained the most advanced level of psychic organization of all pathological entities, and this expresses the adaptive effort to continue the thrust of developmental progression.

When hysterical symptoms are not effective in managing instinctual overstimulation or when there is no oedipal conflict resolution, the fixation points are tenaciously and defensively maintained. They are at the foundation of fixed attitudes designed to protect against genital instinctual overstimulation. The stimuli of the internal and external worlds are then distorted by the influence of these phallically determined memory traces of an infantile attachment to an object and of infantile instinctual experience, and hysterical character pathology is manifsted. All interactions, and all instinctual activity, are perceived and reacted to as having phallic significance. Symptoms form in an open system of perception, whereas character pathology forms in a fixed system of perception. Hysterical character pathology develops as an adaptive response to the anxiety aroused by stimuli evocative of the over-stimulating effects of an unresolved oedipal conflict.

Hysteria has been defined and described throughout the literature in a host of ways. There have been discussions of "good" hysterics and "bad" hysterics and discussions concerning the relationship of orality and genitality. Disorers manifesting distortions in body ego experience can occur at all levels of personality organization. The entire continuum could include the hysterias, the cohesive narcissistic personality disorders, the distortions in self-experience created by splitting mechanisms in the borderline personality, and the bizarre self-experiences seen in the schizophrenias. Hysterical symptom and character pathology involve object-related, intrapsychic conflicts, in a genitally organized personality with repression proper as the major defensive activity of the ego. The most advanced level of personality organization is one in which symptomatic compromises can be formed.

The Obsessive Disorders

Obsessive character pathology is next in the descending order of a developmental hierarchy of diagnostic categories, followed by obsessive symptom formation. Obsessive symptoms are formed when there has been a regressive breakdown in the defensive function of fixed character attitudes. Symptomatic compromises are effected in an open system of perception, to prevent further regression and alleviate the threat of fragmentation.

The association of a genital oedipal conflict coexisting with powerful anal-sadistic components has long been noted in the obsessive disorders. The consistent connection between traits of cruelty and anal erotism was first specifically identified by Jones (1913). Freud (1915/1963) directed attention to the anal-sadistic orientation of the obsessive. These individuals exhibited a constant concern over aggression and submission, cruelty and kindness, duty and cleanliness, order and disorder. Sometimes these characteristics were only seen in reaction formations, such as overkindliness, an exaggerated sense of cleanliness, or an inability to exhibit any signs of aggression. The instinctual organization was described as resembling the child in the anal-sadistic phase of psychosexual development. Anal eroticism has been linked with the obsessive disorders throughout the psychoanalytic literature.

The oedipal conflict is organized at the end of the pahllic phase with a consolidation of the component instincts into a genital drive. The reasons for an apparent anal-sadistic fixation were important to delineate. Generally, it was explained by conceptualizing a regression to this earlier period of difficulty, as a response to oedipal anxieties. Fenichel's (1945) conception was that the defense was first directed against phallic-oedipal conflicts, which instigated a regression. Oedipal wishes were then supplanted with anal-sadistic wishes, and the defenses continued against these anal impulses. Freud (1924/1959) pictured the obsessive as perceiving sexuality in anal terms, as if it were a bathroom affair. The enhanced sadism exaggerated the oedipal rivalries to such an extent that the resulting threat of castration was heightened and a defensive shift was necessary. In the male, this included a shift to the male as a sexual object.

Over the years, it became apparent that the influence of anality was much greater than could be explained by regression alone. The psychic organization of the obsessive manifested the imprint of anally determined qualities that were present in all aspects of instinctual experience. This was particularly true in those displaying the fixed anally determined attitudes of character pathology. Regression was much more in evidence in individuals exhibiting obsessive symptoms. A lack of clarity in distinguishing the relationship of obsessive character pathology with an absence of symptoms, to obsessive pathology with symptoms, tended to obscure this distinction between regression and fixation. In addition, obsessive features are frequently manifested in a wide variety of disorders. The obsessive neurotic disorders are object related and based upon intense oedipal conflicts. When obsessive symptoms are expressed, they are embedded in an obsessive character structure. Individuals with a narcissistic orientation may display obsessive characteristics, but they are intermixed with other aspects of psychic functioning.

Many authors have defined the pathology in the obsessive as an elaboration of compensatory mechanisms. Intellectualization and overideational activities are utilized in an attempt to master the traumatic impact of instinctual demands. The mechanism of isolation, which is essential for the adaptive functions of concentration and logical thinking, is overdeveloped and serves a defensive function. Intellectualization, isolation, and reaction formations are hallmarks of the defensive orientation, and their relationship to repression proper is important to define. Many psychoanalytic clinicians have viewed the use of these defenses as evidence that repression proper is either superfluous, or nonfunctional. The presence of impulse derivatives in consciousness, usually considered to be repressed, is explained as the consequence of these mechanisms not allowing repression to be utilized or as an indication of its deficient functioning. This formulation has led to some confusion in understanding the personality organization of the obsessive and in making a clear diagnosis. In this presentation, the relationship of these mechanisms to repression proper is formulated. Reaction formations are especially significant because they create changes in self-experience from the effects of an object's influence. They represent the beginning stages in the organization of the superego and are interwoven with the functioning of the fixation points. Repression proper is defined as a perceptual activity and requires the structuralization of cohesiveness to be functional. When there is a regressive breakdown in the defensive function of the fixation point on the introjective arm of perception, instinctual derivatives of unconscious mental activity emerge into consciousness and are included in the compromises of obsessive symptoms. Repression proper continues to be operative, but the psychic contents available to be perceived are now different. It is the defensive alignments designed to reenforce repression that are ineffective, rather than the function itself.

Sandler and Joffe (1965) made an effort to explain the regressive functioning of the ego seen in the obsessive, by defining the roles of perception and cognition. These authors pointed out the assumed connection that often exists between drive regression to anal-sadistic fixation points and defenses of isolation and reaction formation. The problem has been that it is a change in the ego that determines the neurosis, at the same time that the mental structures remain unchanged, and they postulated a functional regression of the ego. Defenses in general are adaptations of normal ego functions. The particular type of defensive organization is as crucial to the determination of the form of pathology, as is the fixation and regression. They speculated that this organization is latently present from the point of its formation and is inherent in the particular style of perception and cognition.

In considering obsessive pathology, there has been general agreement in several areas. In relation to the drives, there is a regression to the anal-sadistic level. Marked ambivalence is a characteristic of this pregenital phase and is abundantly evident in the obsessive. The ego displays an increase in magical thinking with a heightened sexual and aggressive cathexis of thought. Defenses of reaction formation, isolation, and undoing are actively present, as are the excessive uses of intellectualization and rationalization. In regard to object relationships, there is never a complete regression to anality. It is an analization of oedipal relationships. The structure of the ego is intact, the ideals of the superego persist, and a defensive struggle is carried on against the drives and their derivatives at a drive-regressed level. The obsessive manifestations frequently seen in borderline and psychotic individuals represent an attempt on the part of the ego to deal with threats of annihilation or fragmentation. The basic anxiety is not primarily from conflict, and the symptoms constitute an effort to achieve a degree of security by magical means. This again emphasizes the importance of the overall psychic organization, rather than the particular symptom, in making a diagnosis.

The fixed character attitudes of the obsessive are formed during the anal phase, influence all further instinctual progression and personality advancement, and hence are evident in childhood. When an obsessive disorder appears later in life, there are many indications of anally fixed character attitudes that have been present since childhood. In addition, these fixed character traits are frequently observed in children. A developmental perspective would anticipate a similarity between their expression in childhood and in the adult. Anna Freud (1966) discussed the resemblance of the true obsessive neurosis in childhood with its adult counterpart. She outlined the initial developmental progression to a comparatively high level of drive and ego development. In the child, the progression extended into the phallic-oedipal situation, and in the adult into a genital configuration. In both child and adult, an intolerable increase in anxiety or frustration led to a regression to pregenital fixation points and the emergence of infantile pregenital sexual and aggressive impulses, wishes, and fantasies. The anxiety and guilt associated with the pregenital drives mobilized defensive reactions under the influence of the superego. The resulting compromise was manifested in a character disorder or a neurotic symptom. The level of the fixation points to which regression had taken place, the content of the rejected impulses and fantasies, and the choice of the particular defense mechanisms determined whether character pathology or symptoms were expressed. She underscored the importance of making a distinction between obsessive manifestations that bear some resemblance in form and content to those of an obsessive neurosis and those that often occur in children during the anal phase of development as a consequence of regression.

Anna Freud (1965) summarized the state of knowledge concerning the obsessive-compulsive neuroses and reflected upon the range of severity. It varied from ego syntonic and near-normal manifestations in character formation to the status of an extremely severe neurotic disturbance bordering occasionally on the schizoid and schizophrenic. On the normal end of the continuum, obsessional manifestations are stabilizing in their effects upon the personality. At the extreme end, they are crippling and harmful for internal equilibrium. The relationship of one to the other end of this continuum has never been adequately explained.

It is my impression that one reason for confusion is the unclear delineation of the manner in which fixation points are formed and the manner in which they function. The id content in obsessional disorders involves impulses of the pregenital anal-sadistic stage, which is a clearly demonstrable clinical phenomenon. The connection to a phallic-genital psychic organiztion has only been explained in relation to regressive phenomena. This relationship is more explicable in individuals displaying obsessive symptoms, but with the fixed anally determined attitudes of character pathology, it is less understandable. When the significance of fixation points is considered from the vantage point of perception, the anal orientation of the obsessive within a genitally structured personality can be more effectively elucidated.

This conception is based upon the role of perceptual processes in activating the representational and organizational functions of the ego. Body ego experiences are registered, coalesce into good and bad entities according to the need for defense, and form a system of self-representations. Their object-impression counterparts are also registered, coalesce into good and bad entities, and form a system of object representations. During the process of separation–individuation, the two systems are connected by the recognition of a separate good object's influence, whiich extends the boundaries of the self. Two arms of perception and a focused area of perceptual activity are formed, establishing the skeletal framework of cohesiveness. An introjective arm of perception represents the extension of self-experience toward perceiving the impressions of a separate good object, a projective arm of perception represents the connection to the system of object impressions, and the focused area of perceptual activity operates as the eye of consciousness enabling the function of self-observation. Initially, cohesiveness is highly unstable, until a fixation point is formed on the projective arm of perception. It is based upon an awareness of the good object's bad prohibitive qualities, anchors object constancy and differentiation, and provides the necessary stability for linking the mental structures that further differentiation. These mental structures, the grandiose self and ego ideal, prepare the groundwork for continuing advancement toward a genital organization. The grandiose self buffers the vulnerability associated with separateness by linking the representation of good instinctual self-experience to a fantasy of a good object's influence. The ego ideal strengthens adaptive functions by including the needed influences of an object within self-experience. This process of selective identification directs perceptual attention into the self-system of representations. A fixation point is then formed on the introjective arm of perception, based upon an awareness of the good self's bad instinctual qualities, which provides the needed stability for the oedipal fantasies to exert their organizing influence. In healthy development, these sequential steps take place in a stage- and phase-specific manner, and with the resolution of the oedipal conflict, the fixation points are freed of their infantile attachments.

The obsessive has advanced developmentally to the formation of an oedipal conflict but has been out of step with stage and phase specificity, has not achieved a resolution of that conflict, and remains under the influence of the infantile attachments at the foundation of the fixation points. Early development has been characterized by an excessive degree of frustration, instigating a somewhat premature process of separation–individuation. The fixation point on the projective arm of perception is formed very early in the anal phase and is based upon the unmodulated impressions of an anally sadistic object. In not being stage and phase specific, the vulnerability associated with separateness is more extreme, and the grandiose self is linked by the fantasy of an anally derived good object's omnipotence that is exaggerated and somewhat unstable. It is with the formation of the ego ideal that the seeds of pathology begin to unfold. The preponderance of anal-sadistic aggression is poorly regulated, which creates the need for the restraining influences of an object. The ego ideal is structured prematurely during the anal phase, by including the prohibitive impressions of an anally sadistic object within self-experience. this is the foundation upon which anally determined reaction formations are constructed and is accompanied by the formation of a fixation point on the introjective arm of perception. This fixation point is based upon an awareness of the good self's bad instinctual qualities, which are the threatening anal-sadistic experiences altered by the prohibitive force of an anally sadistic object's influence. these precociously established fixation points, which serve a defensive as well as a stabilizing function, are tenaciously bound to their original memory traces. A fixed anally determined influence is then exerted upon all further advancement in instinctual representation and upon the stimuli emanating from contact with the external world. Continuing instinctual expansion into phallic and genital dimensions takes place, but with this strong anal coloration. The structure of castration anxiety and the genital fantasies of the oedipal conflict are distorted by the dominant effect of anality, and the demand for severe prohibitions is reflected in the developing superego. Ongoing selective identifications tend to overemphasize the anal attitudes of overcontrol and opposition to instinctual activity, and deficiencies in self-experience are compensated for by overelaborating the representations of the object.

A clear distinction has also not been made between those who present obsessive symptoms embedded in an anally influenced genital character organization and those in which there is a mixed character and symptom picture. The ego devices present in all neurotic obsessive phenomena are repression, anally determined reaction formations, isolation, undoing, magical thinking, doubting, indecision, intellectualization, and rationalization. The characteristic of these ego devices is their overemphasis on the functioning of the thought processes. The clinical picture is shaped primarily by the reaction formations, which give the impression of stability and unalterability. The intensity of countercathexis creates an inner sensation of mental strain, which is added to by the effort to bind id energies through secondary-process thinking. This particular aspect of functioning ties the obsessive disorders to a higher level of ego development. It appears that there is no obsessive neurotic disorder in which reaction formations and intellectualizations do not play a part. This differentiates it from other disorders that on the surface may appear similar but have an entirely different psychic organization. For example, the repetitive tendencies that are manifested in various pathological states, and the compulsivity that seems to govern certain addictions and delinquencies, operate under an entirely different set of principles. The conditions that seem to favor the development of neurotic obsessive pathology involve a precocious maturation of the ego functions and what appears to be an increase in the intensity of anal-sadistic tendencies. Occcasionally, they are associated with traumata during the anal phase, in the form of seductions or interference by excessively strict training. Obsessive individuals are characteristically at cross-purposes with themselves and with objects in the external world. The intrasystemic contradictions of love and hate, activity and passivity, feminity and masculinity, are heightened.

The Narcissistically Determined, Object-Related Disorders: The Phobias

The concept of phobic symptomatology was originally introduced by Freud (1910/1955) to distinguish a neurosis whose central symptom was a phobia and to emphasize its structural resemblance to conversion hysteria. For many years, anxiety hysteria and phobias tended to be utilized as synonymous terms, until it became apparent that phobic symptoms were seen in a variety of pathological states. The original relationship to conversion hysteria was based upon the concept that the task of repression was to effect a separation of affect and idea. This early formulation depicted libido as being converted and expressed in a bodily function in the conversion hysterias and as being set free and expressed in the form of anxiety in the phobias. Fenichel (1945) thought of the phobias as an expression of the body and its sensations that could not be avoided, so that an advantageous projection from an internal instinctual danger to an external perceptual danger took place. The anxiety was avoided by an appropriate phobia, at the cost of the freedom of the ego, and the instinctual danger was turned into a perceptual one. Claustrophobia was conceived of as the fear of one's own excitement, which was projected and externalized. In these early formulations, no distinction was made between phobias that are characterized by avoidance with a limited capacity for instinctual representation, and anxiety that is associated with instinctual representation and the elaboration of fantasy.

In the early psychoanalytic writings, which were replete with acute clinical observations, there were limitations in ego psychological and object relations theory. This necessitated that intricate psychic mechanisms be formulated to explain the psychic contents observed in the phobias. Deutsch (1929), for example, noticed the significance of a companion. The presence of a companion eased the phobic situation in some and did not in others. This was explained on the basis of the companion representing the protecting parent, but also the unconsciously hated parent, and of diverting the patient's mind from unconscious fantasies to reality. Little attention was directed to the particular qualities of the relationship or to the specific representations of self-experience and of an object's influence that were evoked by an interaction. Attention was paid almost solely to the unconscious conflict expressed by the symptom, which tended to ignore the underlying foundations of character from which the symptom emerged.

In this presentation, the underlying psychic organization that determines a phobic attitude is discussed in detail. A distinction is made between phobias, which are founded upon a narcissistic fixation and reflect a threat to cohesiveness, and anxieties, which are founded upon an object-related structural organization and symbolically represent an instinctual danger. It is my impression that the increase in instinctual activity associated with the demands of an oedipal conflict have been overwhelming to the phobic, and it is this developmental step that has not been negotiated. Phobic symptoms are grouped into three categories, which exist on a continuum and fluctuate within a given individual. These include (1) the object phobias, in which the self is symbolically represented as threatened by a devouring monster; (2) the self-phobias, in which the self is symbolically represented as trapped and immobilized within an enclosed space; and (3) the combined self- and object phobias, in which there is little capacity for symbolic representation and the phobic response is to environmental stimuli. The greater the stability of the structures that maintain differentiation and cohesiveness, the more an object phobia is likely to be manifested and the more advancing instinctual representation is in evidence even to the point of a genital consolidation.

Anna Freud (1977) referred to the wide variety of patients who suffer from fears and anxieties. The sources were external as well as internal and defended against by a variety of means, from a primitive need for reassurance to sophisticated obsessional defenses. Phobic avoidance was only one of a multitude of mechanisms. In this article, she described the host of reactions to danger that are derived from all levels. They ranged from the archaic anxiety of annihilation, to separation anxiety, to castration anxiety and guilt. She stressed the unsolved conceptual problems in regard to the phobias. Phobia means avoidance, and there is a gap in the understanding of what determines this specific response. Most individuals deal with anxiety by profuse fantasy activity and use many different defensive means. The construction of a fantasy is aimed at keeping anxiety at a tolerable level. Some authors have indicated that a phobic individual not only flees from the object of anxiety but is fascinated and compulsively drawn to it. She felt this was not borne out by clinical observation because the phobic defense appears to blot out any positive seductive aspect that may be hidden in the anxiety. In the absence of the phobic object, the individual is, in fact, peaceful. What appears to be happening is that the underlying character and personality organization is in a precarious position and easily upset by some ''intrusive event.'' A happening in the external world brings the warded-off danger to the surface and creates a state of panic. The only resort is to flight, by externalizing the source of danger. According to Anna Freud, this formulation ignores the important step of condensation preceding the process of externalization. The fears and anxieties do not remain diffuse but are compressed into one symptom. That symptom represents the dangers of the preoedipal as well as the dominant phallic-oedipal threat, and the symbol is dealt with by avoidance.

Anna Freud (1977) also underscored the importance of viewing the effects of anxiety from two sides. There is a pathogenic aspect and a beneficial unpleasure that are essential for promoting certain developmental steps. Archaic fears lead to a child's clinging to the mother and increase object relatedness. The fear of loss of love and criticism is an important incentive for educational demands. The anxiety aroused by the strength of id impulses furthers the construction of effective defenses. The fear of the superego leads to drive modification and social adaptation. Thus, the same unpleasant affects that cause neurotic symptoms are indispensable assets to promote character building. It is essential to delineate the dividing line between that which is positive and that which is negative and to have a conception of the impact of fear and anxiety. This is particularly demonstrable in the phobic individual, whose reaction to a phobic object is closer to a panic state. It may be that the dreaded confrontation with panic accounts for the use of this most primitive of all defenses. Phobias seen in this light could be understood as an alternative to traumatization.

Avoidance is the special response that characterizes a phobia, which frequently fluctuates and expands. The individual with a phobic symptom has a basic phobic attitude toward inner and outer stimuli, and although the anxiety is of panic proportions, it is only manifested under specific conditions. This latent fixed phobic attitude appears to be a reflection of the underlying character makeup, and when the phobic symptom is present, the predominant anxiety is of the loss of differentiation. It is this quality of the anxiety that calls attention to the narcissistic nature of psychic structuralization. Yet the phobic symptom is indicative of some capacity for symbolization and for progression toward containing instinctual activity through the representation of derivatives. In that respect, the phobia meets some of the criteria for psychological symptom formation. A compromise is effected within the ego, as instinctual activity and defensive opposition are given some expression. This aspect of the phobia has fostered the formulation of its conflictual significance. It appears to me that it is more accurate to conceptualize a progressive movement toward conflict formation. Advances in instinctual representation are excessively traumatic to the psychic organization of the phobic individual, and the response to this danger is a regression to a narcissistic fixation. The specific composition of this narcissistic fixation is the basis for the phobia. Many authors have observed that the acute anxiety comes first and the phobia emerges as a defense.

The anxiety leading to the formation of a phobic symptom is of traumatic proportions, and the threat is to the integrity of the self. This is in contrast to the anxiety associated with the expression of unconscious fantasies and their derivatives. Greenson (1959) hypothesized that the anxiety in the phobias was derived from the terror of psychic helplessness. The phobia is preceded by an acute state of anxiety in which there is a loss of the ego functions of memory, perception, mobility, identity, and body integrity. He referred to the loose connection to any given diagnostic category and noted that they were more likely to occur in an underlying pregenital psychic organization. Greenson considered the predominant anxiety to be the crucial determinant of a diagnostic understanding. Every level of development has its specific fears, and it is the quality of the anxiety rather than the intensity. He speculated that the panic anxiety, observed in the phobias, reflected a threatened loss of the internal cathexis of an object.

Many analysts have suggested there was something specific about a phobic reaction, having significance for understanding a phase in development that had gone pathologically awry. There is general agreement that the core of the experience is in the nature of the anxiety, which is of traumatic proportions. Trauma is determined by two sets of factors: the condition of the ego and the quantity of the stimuli. In the course of healthy development, the consolidation of the component instincts into a genital drive creates a potential state of trauma. This phobic situation is a consequence of the narcissistically structured condition of the ego, in conjunction with an increase in the quantity of instinctual demand. It serves as an impetus for the oedipal conflict to be set in motion, which results in a changed conditon of the ego and an increased capacity for instinctual representation. I have postulated that the phobic disorders are the pathological sequelae of an inability to negotiate this developmental step and are repetitively attempting to master the shift from a narcissistic to an object-related orientation.

The psychic organization of individuals with phobic symptomatology has appeared to me to be identical with those diagnosed as cohesive narcissistic personality disorders. In both, the structures maintaining a narcissistic fixation are similar, and the primary anxiety is of a loss of cohesiveness. In some, phobic symptoms are overt, and in others they are latent. When phobic symptoms are in evidence, they highlight the area of greatest vulnerability, and reflect the degree of progression toward object relatedness. The object phobias display a capacity for instinctual representation, but the elaboration of psychic content in the object system of representations is curtailed. The self-phobias are capable of elaborating the representations of an object, but instinctual experience is inhibited. The combined self- and object phobias display little capacity for elaborating psychic content in either system of representations. The object phobia symbolically represents the threat to cohesiveness by the influences of a bad object, the self-phobia symbolically represents the threat to cohesivenss by instinctual overstimulation, and the combined self- and object phobias are threatened by both. The object phobias show the most progression toward a genital organization and exhibit features similar to the hysteric. The self-phobias are deficient in instinctual representation and exhibit features similar to the obsessive. The combined self- and object phobias are narcissistically fixated and possess characteristics attributable to the narcissistic personality disorders. Although there are some similarities to the hysteric and obsessive, the differences are diagnostically significant. In the phobias, instinctual representation is limited, loss of cohesiveness is the primary threat, and the personality is narcissistically structured. In the hysteric and obsessive, there is a large capacity for instinctual representation, castration anxiety is the primary threat, and the structure of the personality is object related. In the neurotic, hysterical symptoms are manifested upon the substrate of a hysterical character and obsessive symptoms on the substrate of an obsessive character. The phobic shifts from one phobic organization to another, displays a mixed symptom and character picture, and under stress has all of the features of a narcissistic personality disorder. In this presentation, I will formulate the developmental line for the structural foundation of this phenomenon.

Arlow (1963), in discussing the nature of fantasy, pointed out its importance in reflecting the level of ego functioning at the time of the original conflict. The expression of danger is based upon sensory imagery or experience. Fantasies thereby reveal the level of instinctual wishes and also demonstrate the effects of the integrative functions of the ego. The object phobia represents the danger as being the influence of an orally incorporative object. The self-phobia represents the danger as one of being swallowed up by the effects of instinctual overstimulation. The combined self- and object phobias experience vague and ominous threats to the integrity of the self, which reflect orally determined concerns of loss of differentiation. Further exploration into the developmental history of phobic individuals unearthed one striking similarity. This involved an empathic psychological symbiotic period, which was abruptly interrupted by a traumatic change in the conditions of empathy specifically at the point that the process of individuation was beginning to assert its activity. The experience seemed to initiate an extremely premature internal search for a separate good object's influence. Separation–individuation is negotiated during the oral phase, under traumatic conditions, which affects the composition and function of the fixation points and of the structures maintaining cohesiveness. The fixation point on the projective arm of perception, designed to maintain differentiation, is based upon oral incorporative qualities that threaten differentiation. The solution is in a phobic attitude toward the influences of a bad object. The vulnerability of separateness is extreme, and the grandiose self is structured by participation in the fantasy of an orally derived, all-giving nurturer. Adaptive functions are depleted by the relative dearth of good self-experience, and the ego ideal is structured by including the optimally gratifying influences of an orally determined good object within self-experience. The grandiose self and ego ideal are composed of the same aspect of an object's influence, are not well delineated from each other, and function as a unit. The fixation point on the introjective arm of perception is also formed late in the oral phase and is based upon an awareness of oral instinctual experiences that are devouring in nature. They are potentially threatening to cohesiveness and create the readiness to develop a phobic attitude toward instinctual overstimulation. There is sufficient structuralization for some forays into more adanced levels of instinctual representation to occur, even to the point of a genital consolidation. However, the profound influence of orality does not support the demands of an oedipal conflict, and the response is to regress to a previously established narcissistic fixation. The instability of the fixation points, and the fluidity in functioning of the grandiose self and ego ideal, appear to be at the foundation of the shifts from one phobic position to another. This hypothesis seemed consonant with the observations of a number of authors, who pointed to the loose connection of phobias to any diagnostic category. I have conceptualized phobias within a developmental framework, reflecting the transition from a narcissistic to an object-related orientation under the influence of an orally determined character structure. As Greenson (1959) and others have pointed out, it is the quality of the anxiety that is of prime significance in establishing a diagnosis. Castration anxiety predominates in a phallic and genital organization. The anxiety of loss of the object's love and of loss of control characterizes an anal organization. The anxiety of being devoured, or of the loss of ego functions, body integrity, and identity, reflects the influence of orality.

The phobic attitude toward the influences of a bad, orally incorporative object is based upon the fear of losing all functional capacities. The ability to maintain differentiation and cohesiveness is at issue, not necessarily the demand for a compromise solution. The ego, in representing this threat, is offering some degree of containment and regulation. To the extent that the phobic situation is then alleviated, advancing instinctual representation becomes a possibility, and conflict emerges as the primary danger. In a phobic situation, the primary threat is of loss of differentiation, and the need is for avoidance. The phobic situation that developmentally initiates a shift form narcissism to object relatedness is consistent with the almost universal presence of transient phobic reactions in children at precisely this juncture. With the elaboration of genital fantasies and regulatory responses, the phobic situation is alleviated, and instinctual conflict becomes predominant. The quality of the anxiety in the phobias is particularly significant because it is the demands of oedipal conflicts that seem to be so overwhelming. It has been my observation that a phobic situation must be alleviated before phallic and genitally determined conflicts and anxieties are manifested. It also offers an explanation for the frequency with which phobias precede the formation of an obsessional neurosis in children. This is especially difficult to explain when phobias are viewed as the product of a genital conflict. Phobic responses to environmental stimuli, with little overt evidence of their having instinctual meaning, have also required an explanation. The data of a combined self- and object phobia in which cohesiveness is threatened by the influences of a bad object and by instinctual overstimulation, with little capacity for representation, is consistent with this phenomenon. Conceiving of an instinctual danger's being displaced, projected, and externalized to become a perceptual danger, describes the events, but does not explain how a body ego experience can be managed in this way.

Kernberg (1976) reexamined Fenichel's classification of character and defined the structural consequences of pathological object relationshps to the ego and superego. He outlined the three major pathological developments in the formation of character: one, the pathology in the ego and superego structures; two, the pathology in internal object relationshps; and three, the pathology in the development of libidinal and aggressive drive derivatives. In considering these factors, character traits based upon reaction formations are much more advanced developmentally. Those based upon phobic attitudes are more primitive and narcissistically determined. The mechanism of identification with the aggressor, essential for the formation of reactive character traits, is largely unavailable in the phobic individual because the influences of a prohibitive object are orally derived, incorporative in nature, and phobically avoided.

Nagera (1981) addressed the concept of fixation and noted that it had several references. A fixation can refer to a given component instinct, a phase of libidinal and aggressive development, a type of object choice, a type of object relationship, and/or a traumatic experience. Fixation points always indicate some degree of an arrest in development. When a fixation point can encompass so many variables, it accentuates the importance of a concept capable of illuminating the psychological foundation for these different aspects of mental functioning. I have approached it by defining fixation points on the basis of the interrelationship between perceptual processes and the representational functions of the ego. The manner in which stimuli are registered and represented and their effect upon psychic structuralization determine the composition and function of a fixation point. They are formed at two locales. One is in the realm of object impressions, where the awareness of a good object's bad prohibitive qualities anchors object constancy, supports projective processes, and sustains a differentiated connection to the influences of an object. It is founded upon memory traces of an infantile attachment to an object, with qualities dependent upon the phase of psychosexual development in the ascendency at the time of its formation. Initially, it provides the necessary stability for the grandiose self and ego ideal to be structured. The second fixation point is in the realm of self-experience, where the awareness of bad instinctual qualities stabilizes the influx of new stimuli. It is founded upon the memory traces of infantile instinctual experience in the ascendency at the time of its formation. Initially, it is necessary to enable the oedipal conflict to exert its organizing influences without the disruptive effect of incoming stimuli. The fixation points are not necessarily indicative of an arrest in drive development, although their composition reflects and perpetuates such an arrest. They are essential to provide the stability for new structure formation, which furthers differentiation and advances instinctual representation. When the fixation points themselves are unstable, delayed or prematurely formed, or defensively maintained beyond stage and phase specificity, it is the product of an arrest in drive development. In the phobias, the points of fixation are highly unstable because they are based upon the memory traces of an attachment to an object and of instinctual experiences that pose a threat to cohesiveness. The result is in a lack of flexibility that does not facilitate the effective representation of advancing levels of instinctual demand. These points of fixation are defensively maintained, give an oral cast to all stimuli, and do not offer the stability necessary to negotiate the shift from narcissism to object relatedness.

Nagera (1981), in discussing the effects of pregenital fixations, described the pull they exert upon the higher levels of development that are attained. Even slight difficulties at more advanced levels of organization will quickly lead to a regression when these fixation points are an active force. Once the phallic oedipal stage is reached, although a regression may take place, the representations of this advancement remain. The phobias, which are narcissistically determined and object-related disorders, often give evidence of this limited foray into a genital consolidation. However, the full elaboration of an oedipal conflict has not taken place, and a genital object-related organization cannot be sustained.

Nacht (1966) observed that an obsessional neurosis often followed closely on the heels of a phobic neurosis. She pointed out that the defenses and organization of the ego in the obsessive are much more evolved than in the phobic disorders. Phobic attitudes and a phobic organization seemed much closer to the source of trauma, and she directed attention to the effects of unconscious empathic responsiveness in alleviating a phobic situation. Many authors have noted the psychic consequence of traumatic lapses in empathy during critical phases in the early development of individuals with narcissistic disorders. The specific traumata, and the specific phases in which they occur, are often recreated in the transference relationship. When empathic lapses occur, they resonate with the specific mental representations of the developmental trauma. Rothstein (1979) presented examples of patients, identified as narcissistic personality disorders, who had experienced a reality during the course of their development that came close to actualizing what he referred to as their inner oedipal intentions. In this article, he was demonstrating the existence of oedipal factors in narcissistically organized patients and the specific developmental traumata upon which they were based. However, the clinical material reflected an absence of the object-related orientation that is essential for a fully elaborated oedipal conflict to be manifested. Instead, it appeared to be a reflection of the forays into a genital consolidation of the drives that can be expressed in an unconsciously empathic environment. When the conditions of a therapeutic environment are empathically responsive to unconscious communications, the effect is to amplify the representations of a good object's influence, strengthen the stability of the structures maintaining cohesiveness, and alleviate the phobic situation. Advances in instinctual representation are then possible, and the therapist is experienced as an instinctual object. Unempathic responses are evocative to the representations of developmental trauma, threaten cohesiveness by intensifying the influences of a bad object, and create a phobic situation. When the therapist is experienced as a phobic object, it is indicative of a failure in empathy. Attributing the phobic reaction to a transference fantasy distortion would be experienced as an attack and recreate the original trauma. The therapist, in understanding that an empathic lapse has occurred, can rectify the failure, interpret its effects, and reestablish an unconsciously empathic interaction.

Kernberg (1970) put emphasis upon the role of excessive oral aggression in the narcissistic disorders and felt that it resulted in a fusion of ideal self, ideal object, and actual self-images. He did not shed light upon how differentiation could be maintained in those narcissistic disorders in which cohesiveness is established. The developmental line and composition of the mental structures that can accomplish this function need to be clarified. Ideal object images are the fantasy elaborations of the impressions of optimally gratifying good objects, which are structurally linked to the representations of good instinctual self-experience to form the grandiose self. Ideal self-images are the fantasy elaborations of deficient self-potentials, which are structurally linked to the needed impressions of an object to form the ego ideal. The grandiose self and ego ideal function to maintain cohesiveness by uniting and differentiating the self- and object systems of representations. In the object-related disorders, these structures are composed of different aspects of an object's influence, have discrete, clearly distinguishable areas of functioning, and are well defined. In the cohesive, narcissistic disorders, exemplified by the phobias, these unifying and differentiating structures blend into each other. If this phenomenum is thought of as a manifestation of the fusion of self- and object images, it is difficult to see how differentiation is maintained. It is my impression that it is not the result of a fusion of self- and object images but that these differentiating structures are formed with the same aspect of an object's influence. The resulting instability is at the foundation of the inordinate need for external objects to regulate self-esteem, for the ready shifts from one phobic position to another, and for the coexistence of mixed symptom and character constellations.

Kohut (1971) discriminated between the transference neuroses and narcissistic transferences. A transference neurosis is seen in object-related disorders, and castration anxiety is the leading source of discomfort. The fear of loss of love, and loss of the object, are of lesser importance. In narcissistic personality disturbances, fear of loss of the object is primary, and castration anxiety is less of a factor. This difference is a reflection of the structural organization of the personality. In the object-related disorders, cohesiveness is well established at the periphery (at the point of perceptual contact with the external world) and at the interior (the point of perceptual contact with the stimuli of biophysiology). Castration anxiety has consolidated into a regulatory structure, capable of a signaling function. In the narcissistic personality disorders, this level of advancement is only sporadically attained and then only when environmental conditions are empathic. The overwhelming anxiety associated with the elaboration of an oedipal conflict instigates a regressive movement to a narcissistic fixation. The loss of the object is then the most important impending threat.

Wangh (1967) believed there was a need to investigate the imbalance in functional characterological forces behind phobic manifestations. He thought the phobias represented an effort to achieve a redressing of the balance between the structural ingredients of the personality. The therapeutic task was to strengthen the ego's capacity to tolerate anxiety and control impulses. The effect would widen the sense of reality, bolster the sense of identity, and increase the capacity to deal with conflict. Arlow (1963) stressed the importance of not blurring the definition of psychological symptom formation and outlined three aspects of psychological experience that needed clarification.

1. *The nature of the danger situation.* Psychological symptoms require sufficient structuralization for a compromise to be effected between an instinctual drive's forcing its way to substitutive gratification and the efforts of the ego to contain it. Arlow felt that many

had blurred the role of conflict, by removing the nature of the danger from the realm of the instinctual drives and their derivatives.

2. *The effects of regression and of preoedipal influences.* When the ego is opposed to the expression of regessively reactivated instinctual wishes and unable to bar expression to their derivatives, symptoms are formed. Arlow felt it would be an error to minimize the importance of preoedipal factors because they exert a decisive influence on the structuring of the psyche. In addition, by tracing the fantasy embedded in the symptom to its origin, it is possible to determine the immature ego organization that existed at the time the fantasy was formed.

3. *The function of fantasies.* Fantasies demonstrate the effects of the integrative functions of the ego. That is, the fantasy gives expression to the danger in concrete form. The nature of the fantasy reveals the level of the instinctual wish and reflects the level of ego functioning at the time of the original conflict. Arlow made it clear that a considerable degree of development is necessary for the structuring of intrapsychic conflict. Therefore, symptom formation is to be found rather late in the period of infantile sexuality.

Phobias stand at the threshold of this capacity for structuring intrapsychic conflict and effecting the necessary compromises to form a symptom. In their most regressed form, manifested by the combined self- and object phobias, the criteria for psychological symptom formation are not met. The phobia can be best understood as a defense against the trauma of loss of differentiation. However, in its more advanced forms, manifested by the object phobias, the criteria for symptom formation are evolving and reflected in the symbolic representation of the phobic object. This gives credence to the concept of phobias as developmentally fixated in the transition from narcissism to object relatedness.

The formation of a psychological symptom involves a compromise within the ego that allows instinctual discharge and defense, meets the demands of the superego, and includes an adaptive response to the demands of the external world. The phobias reflect an inability to negotiate the transition from narcissism to object relatedness and also the transition toward developing the capacity to effect the compromises of symptom formation. Treatment is only concerned with conflict resolution to a limited extent because the primary focus is on alleviating a phobic situation. When phobias are visualized as symbolically representing threats to cohesiveness and as adaptive responses to unconscious perceptions, they can be utilized as a guide for creating conditions that amplify the representations of a good object's influence. The resulting stability facilitates the capacity for instinctual representation, and the aspect of the phobia that does involve conflict resolution can then become significant. When phobias are seen solely as symbolic derivatives of instinctual activity and the conflicts they engender, the tendency would be to understand the phobia as a projection based upon transference distortions alone.

This volume is devoted to a developmental study of those pathological disorders tht occur once a state of cohesiveness has been established. The further steps, along a descending hierarchy of pathological entities, involve the pathological distortions that have occurred in earlier phases of development prior to the negotiation of separation and individuation. These include the borderline personality, the schizophrenias, and the autistic disorders. They will be discussed in another volume.

CHAPTER 1

The Cohesive Disorders

Introduction

The expression, "It all depends on how you look at it," implies that an experience has a different significance if it is viewed from another perspective. A given stimulus can only be perceived from differing perspectives when there is a capacity to effect differing qualities of perceptions simultaneously. The ability to shift from one perceptual vantage point to another depends upon a psychic organization that can support one view, while retaining the effects and significance of the other. It is a complex perceptual act that can only take place when focused areas of perceptual activity, in continuity with each other, are functional in differing sectors of the personality. This requires the representations of self-experience and the representations of an object's influence to be united and differentiated. A shift in perspective can then occur upon a stable background that maintains a continuity of experience, which reflects the presence of a state of cohesiveness.

A Definition of Cohesiveness

Body ego experiences are represented, coalesce, and consolidate into defined entities in accordance with the presence of defense, to form a functional system of self-representations. A whole good self is composed of the experiences that do not require defense; these include (1) phase-specific instinctual gratification, (2) the activity of autonomous ego functions, and (3) the background object of primary identification. A whole bad self is composed of the experiences that involve defense; these include (1) instinctual overstimulation, (2) sensory deprivations, and (3) reactions to impingement. A line of continuity is present in the realm of instinctual experience, as the mounting intensity gradually mobilizes the need for defense.

The object-impression counterparts are similarly represented, coalesce, and consolidate into defined entities to form a functional system of object representations. A whole good object is composed of impressions that do not elicit defense; these include (1) optimal gratification, (2) optimal frustration, and (3) a transitional object. A whole bad object is composed of impressions that elicit defense; these include qualities that are (1) instinctually overstimulating, (2) depriving, and (3) impinging. A line of continuity is present in the realm of restraining influences of an object, as optimal frustration shades into prohibitions and impingments. These object impressions are registered from independent stimuli occurring at two locales. One is at the periphery as a result of contact with the external world, and the other is at the interior in response to that dimension on the continuum of instinctual demand with the independent qualities of an object. This is the portal of entry of instinctual demand, which creates an impression represented as an instinctually overstimulating object.

Cohesiveness is initiated with the first moment of recognition of a separate good object's influence. This transpires during the process of separation–individuation and reflects the establishment of a differentiated connection between the two systems of representations. Cohesiveness expands the self by including the organized influences of an object within its boundaries. This is accomplished as perception is extended in discovering the representation of a good object, which forms two arms of perception and a focused area of internally directed perceptual activity. An introjective arm is extended from the system of self-representations, and a projective arm connects to the system of object representations. The focused area of perceptual activity is at the foundation of the eye of consciousness and function of self-observation. This initial stage of cohesiveness is extremely unstable and is readily lost, until a fixation point is established on the projective arm of perception. It is based upon perceiving the good object's bad qualities through the line of continuity of prohibitive experience and anchors object constancy. The resulting stability enables structural unions to form that strengthen cohesiveness at the periphery. The recognition of separateness is associated with feelings of helplessness and vulnerability, which motivate a search for the influences of an object capable of balancing the experience. This developmental event emerges when anal experiences of mastery and control are in the ascendency and when the representation of an optimally gratifying anal object is elaborated into fantasies of its omnipotence. This fantasy of an object's omnipotence is linked to the instinctual self-experiences of mastery and control and is structuralized, providing balance for the experience of vulnerability. I have called this structure "the grandiose self" because it involves participation in a fantasy. Its effect is to further unite and differentiate the self- and object systems of representations but at the expense of depleting adaptive capacities. The weakening that results from involvement with fantasy motivates a search for the influences of an object capable of strengthening the self-system. The activities of the autonomous ego functions, represented as facets of good self-experience, are elaborated into fantasies of self-potentials. These fantasies link to the influences of an object that are needed and hence admired; this then enables them to be included within self-experience. This process of selective identification is structured to form the ego ideal, which advances the degree of unity and differentiation between the self- and object systems.

The grandiose self and ego ideal have established cohesiveness at the periphery, but at the interior the two systems of representations are only tenuously united. This point of perceptual contact with the stimuli of biophysiological demands is in the locale occupied by representations of a bad object's influence and of bad self-experience. The line of continuity of instinctual experience is represented as a facet of the good self, shades into bad self-experience as defenses are invoked, and extends to the impressions of a bad instinctual object. This latter aspect is the portal of entry of instinctual demand, is the most highly defended, and connects the self- and object systems in a manner that is unreliable. The constant and disruptive impact of instinctual demand is a threat to cohesiveness during these narcissistic stages of development, and there is a continuing vulnerability to the effects of narcissistic injuries until new structures can be formed to unite the two systems at the interior. The expansion of instinctual representation, embodied in the evolution of the component instincts, has reached the limits of what can be represented and regulated within a narcissistically organized personality. The boundaries of the unconscious system are composed of impingements and the reactions to them, are rigid and fixed, and have little capacity for discrimination. Any significant increase in intensity has to be excluded from representation, and the ability to sublimate and utilize instinctual energy in adaptive and intellectual tasks is limited. The unseen dimensions on the continuum of biophysiologic demand are pressing for perceptual attention and representations, creating a potentially phobic situation. The task is to form new structures that can facilitate a continuing influx of instinctual demand.

When the ego ideal is structured, during the phallic phase, perceptual attention is directed into a self-system of representations. The recognition of the good self's bad qualities, through the line of continuity of instinctual experience, establishes a fixation point on the introjective arm of perception. The resulting stability allows the lines of continuity of instinctual and prohibitive experiences to consolidate into the structure of castration anxiety. The signaling and regulatory functions of this structure are a necessary condition for the genital fantasies of an oedipal conflict to flourish. These genital fantasies of bad self-experience and of a bad instinctual object's influence provide linkages between the two systems that are structured to alleviate the potential trauma. The fixation point on the introjective arm of perception establishes the required stability during the period of time that these new structures are formed. The consequence is in a more advanced level of psychic organization, with cohesiveness ensured at the interior of the personality.

Incestuous fantasies, elaborated from the representations of bad genital instinctual self-experience, are linked to the impressions of a bad instinctual object (the portal of entry of instinctual demand). This linkage is structured to establish a new boundary for the unconscious system. It is a reactive, nonperceptual boundary flexible enough to facilitate the elicitation of derivatives in a preconscious system. The prohibitive qualities associated with this union mobilizes defensive responses that enhance its effectiveness in regulating a structured pathway for instinctual integration.

Primal scene fantasies, elaborated from the representation of a bad genital instinctual object, are linked to the representations of self-experiences of genital overstimulation. This linkage is structured to insure a continuous influx of instinctual demand into the self-system. This new structure establishes a pathway of instinctual integration, from the portal of entry of instinctual demand to the self-system of representations, where there is access to attaining secondary autonomy. The selective identifications utilized in resolving the oedipal conflict strengthen the functional capacities within the self-system, enabling instinctual demand that had previously required defense to be included as a facet of good self-experience. This process dissolves the fixation point on the introjective arm of perception and completes the pathway of instinctual integration. Instinctual demand, in traversing this pathway, has attained secondary autonomy and is available as an inner boundary for the conflict-free sphere of the ego. This sector of conflict-free functioning is organized into a system, which acts in harmony with the superego to guide continuing self-expansion. Cohesiveness is secured throughout the personality, the fixation point on the introjective arm of perception is relinquished, and there is sufficient structuralization and internal regulation for the self to be enhanced through object-related experiences.

The Significance of Object-Related Perceptions

During the narcissistic phases of development, the object's importance is determined by the qualities that are brought to enhance self-experience. Orally, it involves incorporative experiences; anally, the opportunities for mastery and control; phallically, the reflection of exhibitionistic activities. This is as far as instinctual representation can expand with a narcissistic orientation. Continued expansion cannot take place until there is a shift in attitude, in perception, and in self-experience. The consolidation of the component instincts into a genital drive is associated with an increase in intensity of instinctual demand, which cannot be represented by narcissistically determined structures. The phobic situation motivates the flowering of an oedipal conflict that exerts an organizing influence upon the personality. The genital is established as the symbolic organ of connection to an object, and the genital fantasy elaborations that comprise the oedipal conflict form new structures that enable the shift from narcissism to object relatedness. These new structures are at the foundation of the capacity to register and represent the unseen dimensions of instinctual demand, and associated with it, the capacity to perceive an external object as having unseen, independent objects of its own. This object-related perception, in a narcissistic state, was experienced as an impingement that had to be defensively excluded from representation. The point at which narcissism shifts to object relatedness is a point at which an increase in instinctual demand or adaptational stress is potentially fragmenting to the continuity of self-experience, unless higher levels of psychic organization evolve. The shift to an object-related orientation creates the ability to ''look'' at the chasm of instinctual demand that has been unseen. The representation of this unseen dimension, through genitally determined primal scene fantasies, allows greater intensities of instinctual demand to be included within self-experience. The oedipal fantasies have exerted an organizing influence upon the personality, creating a shift to an object-related perspective, insured cohsiveness, increased the capacity for instinctual representation, and alleviated the phobic situation.

The resolution of the oedipal conflict strengthens the adaptive integrative capacities of good self-experiences through selective identifications, which are associated with a consolidation of the influences of an object into an independently functioning superego. Instinctual activity that had previously been experienced as overstimulating can be represented without the need for defense, and a continuing influx of instinctual demand is accessible to sublimation and secondary autonomy along a regulated, structured pathway. The conflict-free sphere is organized into a system of ego functions acting in harmony with the functions of the superego. A foundation is established for the gradual disengagement from attachments to the infantile representations of an object and to replace them with the representations of new and independent objects. The perceptual orientation is no longer narcissistic, and the object has shifted in its importance. Self-expansion can continue, enhanced by the ability to experience love for the object.

Cohesiveness is initiated with the first connection of the self- and object systems of representation and is furthered by the formation of unifying and differentiating structures at the periphery. However, it is not ensured until object relatedness is solidly established. There is then sufficient structuralization to heal the early splits in the self that occupy the deepest layers of the id of the dynamic unconscious. These splits have been created by the impact of biophysiological demand upon an immature psychic organization, in the earliest phases of development. The new structures formed by the oedipal conflict not only secure cohesiveness at the interior but also make it possible to absorb and represent the full impact of instinctual demand. When the defensive reaction to this impact is such that it is made inaccessible to representation, the results are in ''blind'' spots and in limitations to the degree of self-expansion that is possible.

The Development and Function of Fixation Points

A fixation point signifies that memory traces have influenced perception, so as to stabilize it and anchor it to the effects of the representations embodied in the memory. Fixation points are essential to provide the stable background necessary for new structures to form and to support object constancy. The internal search for the represented impressions of a good object's influence is the intrapsychic manifestation of the process of separation–individuation. The connection that is made in extending self-experience, to attain a recognition of a separate system of object imagos, forms two arms of perception. One, the introjective arm, is an extension of the self-system of representations. The other, the projective arm, extends to the object system of representations. Fixation points are formed at these locales, in a stage- and phase-specific manner, to facilitate advances in psychic organization.

The first fixation point is formed on the projective arm of perception (where the influences of an object have been represented) to maintain differentiation. During the symbiotic period, the lack of differentiation facilitates the buildup of good self-experience. A system of self-representions is organized into discrete entities of good and bad self-experiences, as their object-impression counterparts are coalescing. Separation–individuation is initiated when good self-experience is sufficiently structuralized to enable the internal search for a good object's influence. The object-impression counterpart of the background object of primary identification is represented as a transitional object. It serves as the nidus around which the other good qualities of optimal gratification and optimal frustration coalesce. When the perception of this representation of a separate whole good object is first attained, it is easily lost. There is a ready return to the undifferentiated fusion and merger experiences of a good object's influence under any conditions of stress or fatigue. The fluctuation continues because the ability to maintain a differentiated view of the object depends almost entirely upon the activity of the autonomous ego function of perception. However, the impressions of an object possessing bad qualities have also coalesced and are accessible to awareness through the line of continuity of prohibitive experience. The recognition of these bad qualities has the effect of fixing the perception of the object as separate. It is not possible to merge with a good object as long as an awareness of its bad qualities is sustained. The memory trace of this infantile attachment to an object establishes a point of fixation on the projective arm of perception.

The function of this fixation point is to stabilize the representations of the object as separate, so that further representation and structure building are able to continue without the severely limiting conditions of a symbiosis. The image of an object can be sustained in the absence of an external object and the presence of frustration, as object constancy is anchored. The experience of vulnerability and helplessness, associated with the recognition of separateness, motivates the formation of the first mental structure that unites and differentiates the two systems of representations. This structure, the grandiose self, utilizes the fantasied omnipotence of an object to gain a sense of balance. The resulting depletion in adaptive capacities is the impetus for forming another unifying and differentiating structure—the ego ideal. This structure includes the needed and admired qualities of an object's influence within self-experience, which forms a pathway for ongoing selective identifications.

The introjective arm of perception has remained open, during these narcissistic phases of development, to enable the internalization of the new experiences necessary to fully negotiate the process of separation–individuation. The ego ideal is structured as instinctual representation has focused upon phallic experiences and as the limits for continuing expansion within a narcissistic organization are being approached. The formation of this structure directs perceptual attention to the self-system of representations, and the line of continuity of instinctual experience is registered. The memory trace of this infantile instinctual experience establishes a fixation point on the introjective arm of perception, based upon a recognition of the good self's bad qualities. The function of this fixation point is to stabilize the influx of new stimuli sufficiently, so that further structural unification can be accomplished without undue interference from its effects.

The lines of continuity of prohibitive experience and of instinctual experience are consolidated to form the structure of castration anxiety. This structure is capable of signaling the need to institute defense and of a variety of regulatory responses from gentle retraint to extremes of prohibition. In conjunction with the stabilizing presence of a fixation point on the introjective arm of perception, the necessary conditions are established for the genitally determined oedipal fantasies to exert their organizing influence. With the resolution of the oedipal conflict, the fixation point on the introjective arm of perception is integrated and relinquished, creating an openness to new experiences from an object-related perspective. The fixation point on the projective arm of perception must remain to anchor object constancy and support projective mechanisms but undergoes a process of depersonification to gradually diminish the effects of narcissistically determined attachments to an object.

The Object-Related Neurotic Disorders: Hysteric and Obsessive Pathologies

Hysteric and obsessional forms of pathologies occur in individuals who have managed to negotiate early developmental tasks and have been unable to negotiate a successful resolution of an oedipal conflict. Cohesiveness and continuity of experience have been well established in the personality, and the component instincts have consolidated into a genital drive. However, the composition of the self- and object systems of representations reflects the imbalances and lack of synchrony in stage and phase specificity that have characterized the narcissistic phases of self-expansion. This, in turn, has had an effect upon the particular infantile attachments to an object and the infantile experiences embodied in the fixation points and upon the functions of the grandiose self and ego ideal. In addition, it affects the manner in which the oedipal fantasies are elaborated and in the inordinate degree of conflict that is engendered. It also has a significant impact upon the process of resolution and shapes the functioning of the superego. The object-related perceptions that have evolved, rather than serving as a source of self-enhancement, are over-stimulating and a source of potential trauma.

The resiliency and viability of the thrust for growth are reflected in the amount of developmental progression that can take place even in the presence of unempathic responsiveness. The developing infant's capacity to attain what is needed from relationships, containing elements that are highly destructive, is often evidenced by the advanced levels of psychic structuralization that are manifested in neurotic pathology. Conversely, an adequate environment often results in neurotic distortions of the developmental process, due to the intensity of instinctual demands and the complexity of the stimuli acting upon an immature psyche. In any determination of causality, it is important to keep in mind that pathological distortions represent an intricate interrelationship between the particular genetic makeup of the individual and the nature of the environment. Phase and stage specificities are vital aspects in the formation of mental structures, and there is such a complex interweaving of internal and external forces that enhance or interfere with that process that there is not a simple one-to-one relationship of causative factors. We can only attempt to define the processes and mechanisms involved in development and the consequences that result from their activity.

The events leading up to the formation of an oedipal conflict determine the particular manner in which it is experienced and represented. In the hysterias, early development has been characterized by libidinal overstimulation. The instinctual impressions of a good object are overdeveloped with an emphasis on orality, optimally frustrating impressions are minimal, and the qualities of a transitional object are sufficient for the advanced structural foundation of an oedipal constellation to evolve. Orality is accentuated; there is a delay in negotiating separation–individuation; and the grandiose self is formed early in the phallic period. In health, the experience of vulnerability associated with separateness occurs during the anal phase. It is perfectly balanced by participating in the fantasied omnipotence of an optimally gratifying object. In the hysteric, the experience of vulnerability associated with separateness occurs when the optimally gratifying impression of an object is elaborated into the fantasy of an admiring audience. The balancing structure of the grandiose self is then based upon participating in the object's admiration rather than omnipotence. The ego ideal forms later in the phallic period, when the developing hysteric is in a state of phallic overstimulation. The qualities of an object that are needed, admired, and selected for identification are those that provide a restraining influence. The impressions of an optimally frustrating object are only minimally represented and do not offer sufficient restraint. Thus the phallically determined impinging and humiliating qualities of a bad object are selected for identification. This has the effect of consolidating the prohibitive function of the superego within the realm of self-experience, eliciting a humiliating response to phallic instinctual activity.

The consolidation of the component instincts into a genital drive and the elaboration of oedipal fantasies take place under conditions of inordinate conflict. The shift to an object-related orientation is accomplished, as new structures are formed for a boundary of the unconscious system and a pathway of instinctual integration. However defensive responses predominate; the boundary of the unconscious system is overdeveloped; and the resolution of the oedipal conflict is inadequate and incomplete. There may be some degree of oedipal conflict resolution, and with it a degree to which the fixation point on the introjective arm of perception is relinquished, but the resulting object-related experiences are overstimulating. Symptomatic compromises are effected to serve a regulatory function, and when they are ineffective, the fixation point is defensively maintained. The consequence is manifested in the fixed attitudes expressive of hysterical character pathology.

The obsessive has had a different set of developmental events leading up to the formation of an oedipal conflict. The degree of frustration during the period of orality has been inordinate and accompanied by a high level of sensory stimulation in other than the instinctual realm. The overabundance of aggression motivates a somewhat premature process of separation–individuation. The grandiose self is structured very early in the anal period, which is close to the situation in healthy development, but the experience of vulnerability is intensified, the omnipotence more extreme, and the stability of this differentiating structure diminished. At this point, the effects upon developmental progression become more accentuated. The ego ideal is structured prematurely, during the anal period, and the fixation point on the introjective arm of perception is also established during this same anal phase. The qualities of an object most admired are those that most effectively restrain the overloading of aggression. Although optimally frustrating influences of an object are abundant and accessible, they do not have sufficient force to regulate the intensity of anal sadistic self-experiences. The prohibitive influence of an anally sadistic object is thus selected, and the resulting identification with a sadistic aggressor elicits a harsh punitive response to any expression of aggression. The reaction formations that are created predominate, as a character fixation is formed early in childhood that influences all further instinctual expansion. Phallic and genital body ego experiences are affected by this anal influence, which shapes the structure of castration anxiety and the emerging oedipal fantasies.

The developing oedipal conflict organizes new object-related structures at the interior, which are a continuous source of potential trauma. The memory traces of anally determined infantile attachments to an object and anally determined infantile instinctual experiences, at the foundation of the fixation points, remain unchanged. The oedipal conflict is incapable of a resolution, and the superego remains in opposition to the interests of the ego, polarized in its functions, and at an immature level of organization. The fixed attitudes expressive of obsessive character pathology are defensively maintained. Symptomatic compromises are only formed when there is a regressive breakdown of the fixation point on the introjective arm of perception.

The Narcissistically Determined Object-Related Disorders: Phobic Pathology

The phobic individual has had an effective psychological symbiosis. It is specifically at the point that separation–individuation is initiated that there is a dramatic change in the experience of empathic responsiveness. The source of that change may be internal or external. The consequence is in an acceleration of the process of separation–individuation, which is set into motion at a very premature period of time. In occurring during the oral phase, they present a number of difficult dilemmas. The impressions of a good object are not effectively differentiated from the body ego experiences of fusion and merger and threaten the tenuously established state of differentation. The line of continuity of prohibitive experience extends to the impression of a bad orally determined impinging object, which is a devouring imago. Thus the fixation point that is established on the projective arm of perception is based upon a recognition of the good object's orally incorporative bad qualities. There is an inadequate distinction between the effects of an object's good and bad qualities, and any awareness of bad qualities is reacted to by a phobic avoidance. The restraining influences of an object are thus of little value in managing and regulating self-experiences of instinctual activity.

An effective symbiotic interaction has changed abruptly at the point that individuation has become viable, which instigates a premature internal search for the influences of a good object. The vulnerability associated with the recognition of separateness is enormous. The grandiose self is structured to balance that experience by linking to the fantasy elaborated from the impression of a good instinctual object, which in the oral phase is of an all-giving nurturer. The resulting depletion in adaptive capacities motivates an urgent need for the strengthening influences of an object, and the ego ideal is structured at a time when there is little available to buffer the impact of narcissistic injuries. In this situation, the optimally gratifying impressions of an object are most admired and selected for identification. The structures of the grandiose self and ego ideal are thereby composed of the same aspect of an object and do not have the differentiated functioning that is present in health and in the neurotic.

The grandiose self is an instinctual structure, uniting and differentiating the self- and object systems of representations. The impetus for its formation is founded upon instinctual self-experience's seeking an object for attachment. In healthy development, this occurs during the anal phase, when instinctual experiences of mastery and control are at their height and the impressions of an optimally gratifying object are elaborated into fantasies of omnipotence. It is this fantasy that makes the structural linkage and provides a perfect match for the vulnerability associated with separateness. Once the two systems are structurally united and differentiated, the conditions are present for the influences of an object to be included within self-experience through a process of selective identification. The depletion in adaptive functions created by participation in a fantasy motivates the formation of the ego ideal, a structure based upon identifications. Self-potentials, reflecting deficiencies in self-experience, are elaborated into fantasies that are linked to the influence of an object that is needed and admired. In health, and in the neuroses, the restraining, regulatory influences of an object are needed, admired, and selected for identification in forming the ego ideal. Thus the two major differentiating structures utilize differing aspects of an object's influence. They function in relation to each other but are not directly concordant. The grandiose self, based on participation in a fantasy, regulates the activities of the primary process; the ego ideal, based upon the influences of external reality, regulates the activities of the secondary process.

In the phobic disorders, the grandiose self and ego ideal are composed of the same representation of the object, the degree of instability is enormous, and the two structures are interchangeable and fluid in their functioning. The fixation points on the projective and introjective arms of perception, which have been formed by a recognition of the lines of continuity of prohibitive and instinctual experiences, are orally determined and based on a phobic avoidance. The distinction between good and bad qualities in the self and object is abrupt. In health, and in the neruoses, the lines of continuity of experience are gradual shadings. Instinctual activity is ineffectively regulated and the restraining force of an object is not available because bad qualities are phobically avoided. Cohesiveness is established but with a very narrow range for the representation of instinctual demand. Instinctual expansion into anal, phallic, and genital body ego experiences may occur, but it is poorly regulated and potentially traumatic and fragmenting. The increase in instinctual demand associated with a genital consolidation and the elaboration of an oedipal conflict is especially threatening.

The differentiating structures of the grandiose self and ego ideal, functioning as one, allow transient shifts from a perceptual focus upon one system of representations to the other. When the focus of perceptual attention is on the influences of an object, the phobic response to bad qualities can be included within self-experience. The extreme tension accompanying the phobic avoidance of bad instinctual self-experience is temporarily alleviated; there is then room for some degree of expansion in the self-system; and the impression of a bad object is represented as a monster threatening the self. This takes place on an unstable background, and any stimulus evocative of a phobic object instigates a shift of perceptual attention into the self-system. The phobic response to bad instinctual experience is represented within the object system as claustrophobia. Under stress, a phobic avoidance is present in both systems, the capacity for representation is limited, and a combined self- and object phobia is manifested in vague, ominous phobic responses to environmental stimuli such as storms, noises, and darkness. In a given individual, these fluctuations from one phobic position to another occur in response to the particular internal and external conditions that are present.

Although limited, some degree of expansion of the component instincts can be represented. This is particularly true when the external world is empathic and nonimpinging. However, the consolidation of the component instincts into a genital drive is associated with an increase in the intensity of instinctual activity that places an overwhelming demand on the phobic individual. This is the underlying anxiety that triggers a narcissistic regression and fixation. In health, and in the neuroses, the fixation point on the introjective arm of perception provides the necessary stability for oedipal fantasies to form new structures. These structures function to insure cohesiveness and increase the capacity for instinctual representation. The capacity for instinctual representation is limited within a narcissistic organization, creating a phobic situation. When the shift from narcissism to object relatedness takes place, the phobic situation is alleviated as the oedipal conflict flourishes. This is the developmental step that the phobic individual has been unable to negotiate. Hysteric and obsessive disorders are disturbances in the development of object relatedness. The narcissistically determined object-related disorders (the phobias) are disturbances in the shift from narcissism to object relatedness. The hysterias and obsessives have developed an oedipal conflict that has been unsuccessfully resolved. The phobias have found the oedipal conflict an overwhelming experience, and the narcissistic fixation is a regression from the demands and threats of object relatedness. It is for this reason that I have called phobias narcissistically determined and object related. It has also appeared to me that the combined self- and object phobias manifest the psychic organization often referred to as narcissistic personality disorders. In the phobic disorders, genital fantasies cannot flourish, the fixation points do not provide sufficient stability to allow an increase in instinctual demand without trauma, the new structures formed by the oedipal conflict are unable to form, and a narcissistic regression is fixated and maintained. The movement is toward object relatedness, but the fixation is narcissistic.

The phobias are often conceptualized as symptomatic expressions of an oedipal conflict. The expectation would then be for the therapist to emerge as a phobic object in the transference, and his task is to interpret the distortions created by the oedipal fantasies. When it is approached in this manner, the effect is to create a temporary or permanent disruption in the treatment as the therapist is phobically avoided. In this formulation, when the therapist is experienced as a phobic object, it is indicative of a lapse in empathy. A therapeutic interaction that is empathic to unconscious communications elicits the functioning of the healthy structures that had been profoundly traumatized by the events of early development. Unconsciously empathic interpretive responses possess the qualities of good objects, which are evocative of these early representations of good self-experience and of good objects' influences. The result is in alleviating the phobic situation and facilitating the progression toward advances in instinctual representation. The therapist is then experienced as an instinctual object, and the associated anxiety is not of phobic proportions.

The qualities of a good object include those of optimal gratification, optimal frustration, and of a transitional object. In a therapeutic interaction, *optimal gratification* refers to the gratification of those aspects of experience that facilitate growth, mastery, autonomy, and independence; *optimal frustration* refers to the abstinence from participating in the reinforcement of pathological defenses; and the *qualities of a transitional object* refers to the therapist's capacity to foster the unfolding of the relationship according to the dictates of an individual's character.

CHAPTER 2

Hysterical Symptom Formation and Hysterical Character Pathology
Preoedipal Determinants

Introduction: Symptom Formation

A psychological symptom is the end result of a series of compromises effected by the ego in an effort to regulate instinctual demands. One aspect of the compromise embodies the interrelationship of id and ego. Instinctual activity pressing for perceptual attention mobilizes defensive responses in opposition to it. The instinctual demand is symbolically represented and hence disguised and modified in its intensity through the defensive functions of the ego. It can then emerge within the realm of preconscious and conscious experiences, where the particular form the symptom takes is shaped and further modified by the compromises necessary in the interrelationship with the superego and with the adaptive demands of the external world. The discomfort created as a consequence of the prohibitive function of the superego is a manifestation of the compromise with the repressive influence of this regulatory agency. The discomfort is proportional to the degree the prohibition is effective and the particular form it takes is determined by the nature of the symptom, the level of organization of the superego, and the perceptual structures that register the disguised instinctual expression. The superego response may thus elicit guilt, shame, or the anxiety of anticipated disapproval. The final compromise is made with the adaptive demands of the external world and is reflected in the secondary gain afforded by the symptom. This refers to its effects upon external objects, which are designed to reinforce the defensive functions of the symptom and simultaneously grant some instinctual expression in action and behavior.

This definition of a psychological symptom gives a generalized overview of the mechanism of symptom formation. The same principle is at work in the process of play and the formation of derivatives, in which the ego's capacity to effect compromises and modify instinctual representation allows the expression of unconscious wishes. In this chapter, I will discuss the conditions that are necessary for hysterical symptoms to occur and the motives and lines of development that eventuate in their formation. I will also attempt to clarify the similarities and differences between hysterical symptom formation and hysterical character pathology, the interrelationship between hysterical symptoms and hysterical character attitudes, the significance of characterological distortions, and the factors that determine the particular nature of a hysterical symptom.

The Fixation Points in the Development of the Hysteric

The preoedipal determinants of hysterical pathology have primarily centered around the consequences of an excessive amount of libidinal overstimulation during the oral phase, with a sufficiency of optimal frustration and ego maturation to achieve separation–individuation, establish cohesiveness and continuity of experience within the personality, and negotiate the shift from narcissism to object relatedness. However, the libidinal overinvolvement with the primary love object has created a significant delay in the movement toward individuation. The recognition of a separate good object's influence does not transpire in a stage- and phase-specific manner, when anal experiences of mastery and control predominate and the fantasy of an object's omnipotence is available to provide a perfect match for the vulnerability associated with separateness. In the developing hysteric, this recognition does not occur until instinctual expansion has reached the phallic phase when the focus of attention is upon body ego experiences of phallic exhibitionism. The extensive engagement with orally determined, libidinal interactions has delayed the full awareness of the good object's bad qualities, which is essential for stabilizing differentiation and the separateness of the self and object. The formation of a fixation point on the projective arm of perception is thus delayed, which is reflected in the particular bad qualities of the object that are perceived. The line of continuity of prohibitive experience, extending from optimal frustration as an aspect of a good object's influence through prohibitions to the impinging impressions of a bad object, has a phallic emphasis. Optimally frustrating impressions of an object are sparse, phallic humiliating impressions abound, and the fixation point that is established bases differentiation upon these phallic impinging attachments to an object.

Another intrapsychic consequence of the prolonged period of libidinal overstimulation, in the early phases of development, is in the plethora of orally derived representations of self-experience and of an object's influence. These dominate in the hierarchal organization of the id of the dynamic unconscious. It is this area of mental activity that exerts an influence on instinctual demands as they are represented along the pathway toward integration. The hysterically predisposed individual exhibits the effects of this excess in orally determined experience, which is manifested in the formation of instinctual derivatives. It is the foundation for the evidences of orality in the phallically determined pathology of hysteria.

The specific nature of the vulnerability and helplessness that is associated with the recognition of separateness depends upon the body ego experiences that are highlighted at the time. When the focus is upon phallic exhibitionism, vulnerability centers upon being humiliated and exposed as inadequate. This is the motive that instigates a search for a linkage to those influences of an object capable of balancing the experience, which is then structuralized to form the grandiose self. The good instinctual impressions of an object are elaborated into fantasies of an admiring audience during the phallic period, and the grandiose self is founded upon admiration rather than omnipotence. The depletion in adaptive capacities, by virtue of participation in this fantasy, motivates the structuralization of the ego ideal late in the phallic period. The composition of this structure is affected by the inadequate regulation of phallic instinctual experience and is accompanied by a recognition of the good self's bad instinctual qualities. A fixation point is then established on the introjective arm of perception that is founded upon the representation of instinctual experiences that quickly move from exhibitionism to voyeurism. The hysteric does not have a balanced progression in the representation of developmental experience or a stage- and phase-specific sequence in the preoedipal structuralization of the personality. Instead, there is an overloading of early oral experiences serving as a background for the phallically determined structures that exert their effects upon the perception of all stimuli.

The Grandiose Self and Ego Ideal in the Hysteric

The delay in initiating the process of separation–individuation has a profound effect upon the composition of the mental structures that are formed to unite and differentiate the self- and object systems of reprsentations. These structures—the grandiose self and ego ideal—are established in response to conditions that are not synchronous with stage and phase specificity. When development proceeds in an orderly sequence, there is a meshing of the stages of instinctual expansion with the formation of mental structures that is perfectly suited to meet a developmental need. The fixation point on the projective arm of perception stabilizes a differentiated connection to the influences of a good object, which enables linkages to be structured between the two systems. The delay in establishing this fixation point has resulted in the representation of instinctual experiences without the restraining influences of an object. The line of continuity of instinctual experience is poorly regulated, so that phallic exhibitionistic activities represented as a facet of good self-experience rapidly become overstimulating and shift to the voyeuristic activities represented within bad self-experience.

The vulnerability associated with separateness is colored by the phallic exhibitionistic experiences that are in the ascendency and takes the form of being humiliated at the exposure of inadequacies. During the phallic period, the impression of a good instinctual object is of delighting in and reflecting back these exhibitionistic activities. A fantasy of an admiring audience is elaborated, which serves as a link that provides balance and is structuralized. The two systems are then united and differentiated by a grandiose self based upon participation in a fantasy of the object's admiration. The readiness with which exhibitionistic experiences become overstimulating places the stability of this structure in jeopardy, which increases the dependency upon external objects for reinforcement. The structured linkage of good instinctual experience by a fantasy has an effect on the self-system of representations. The proportional relationship between good instinctual experiences and bad instinctual experiences is disturbed, and the adaptive functions are diminished. A motive arises to search for, and select, the influences of an object that can be included within self-experience to restore regulation and strengthen functional capacities. The linkage that is established is structured to form the ego ideal.

Optimally frustrating qualities in an interaction have the effect of amplifying autonomous functions and strengthening the resources within the self that foster regulation. The hysteric has moved from experiencing too little optimal frustration to requiring too much self regulation, as instinctual representation has advanced through oral and anal to phallic dimensions. This has a powerful impact upon the qualities of an object's influence that are needed, admired, and selected for identification. The state of phallic instinctual overstimulation dictates a search for the impressions of an object that can provide regulation and restraint. The optimally frustrating impressions of a object, which have a restraining influence, are both deficient and not sufficiently powerful to be effective. The force of impingements are required and perceptually accessible through the line of continuity of prohibitive experience. The deficient self-regulatory functions are elaborated into fantasies that link to the impressions of a phallically impinging object and include this influence within self-experience. This process of identification with an aggressor is structured to form the ego ideal in the hysteric and is the pathway by which the prohibitive force of a humiliating object is carried to the system of self-representations. As a consequence, the readiness for overstimulation has been altered to a constant state of potential humiliation.

Each time exhibitionistic activities become overstimulating and voyeuristic experiences threaten to emerge, the experience available to be registered perceptually is of humiliation. The instinctual experience of exhibiting phallic attributes to an object does not require defense, but as the intensity mounts and defenses are instituted, the excitement shifts to the forbidden act of observing the sexuality of an object. This voyeuristic activity is not actively experienced in the hysteric because it invokes the identifications with a humiliating aggressor and is registered as an object observing the self in a humiliating fashion. (The voyeur, who has the active experience of excitement in observing the sexuality of an object, has an entirely different personality organization and is not hysteric.) This reaction formation is an important aspect of the hysteric's developmental background.

The Nature of Reaction Formations

Phallic exhibitionism is enhanced by the optimally gratifying responses of an empathic external object. These object impressions are represented and elaborated into fantasies of an admiring audience, which forms the linkage that structures the grandiose self. In individuals with a propensity for hysterical pathology, instinctual expressions of phallic exhibitionism were not responded to with a sufficiency of optimal restraint. The influences of an optimally frustrating object offer protection from the potential for humiliation and encompass encouragement to direct these expressions of phallic exhibitionism into channels that do not result in overstimulation. These optimally frustrating qualities of an object are sparsely represented, and the line between optimal restraint and phallically determined humiliating impingements is very thin. The structure of the ego ideal has had to utilize the restraining influences of humiliating impingements to strengthen the capacity to regulate phallic overstimulation in the realm of self-experience. In addition, the consolidation of the component instincts into a genital drive is associated with a high level of instinctual activity evoking the necessity for a powerful prohibitive force. This process of identification with a phallically humiliating aggressor changes the perception of instinctual overstimulation in the self-system of representations and is the basis for the reaction formation that is created.

The grandiose self, ego ideal, and fixation points have all formed during the phallic period, giving a phallically determined meaning to all perceptual contacts. The line of continuity of instinctual experience is poorly regulated, and a demand for perceptual attention is constantly exerted by representations of voyeuristic activity. This serves as a motive to include, within self experience, the prohibitive influences of an object that are in proportion to the intensity of the demand. Phallic instinctual activity involves exposure. Within good self-experience, it is represented as the self exposed to a reflective and appreciative object, and as the intensity mounts, defenses are instituted. An attempt is made to manage the overstimulation by projection, which is manifested as a shift in interest to the sexuality of the object. This forbidden voyeuristic experience reflects a continuing state of overstimulation and requires an additional defensive response. The ego ideal has structured a pathway to the prohibitive influences of an object, which when included within self-experience exposes voyeuristic activities to the impinging qualities of humiliation. Curiosity is a perceptual activity that does not require defense, is a reflection of the utilization of autonomous ego functions, and only invokes a humiliating response when infused with the effects of instinctual overstimulation.

Humiliation is represented as the self in a subservient position, helpless and vulnerable to the narcissistic injury of being exposed as inferior or damaged. The experience of phallic exhibitionism to a reflective audience changes as the intensity mounts. The paucity of restraint for containing and regulating the excitement results in a state of overstimulation, and identifications with a phallic aggressor are invoked. The audience is then represented as disapproving and humiliating, and the self as vulnerable and helpless. The resulting reaction formation places the developing hysteric in a constant state of potential humiliation, which surfaces whenever voyeuristic activities threaten to emerge. The overstimulation associated with the awareness of an object's sexuality is thereby maintained in repression. The experience of self-enhancement through phallic exhibitionism changes to feeling exposed and humiliated, as instinctual experience shifts from exhibitionism to voyeurism. The perception of this overstimulating instinctual activity changes when a reaction formation is established, by a process of identification with a phallic aggressor, and when perceptual attention is focused upon the experience of humiliation.

The Preconditions for a Genital Organization and Their Effects upon the Oedipal Conflict

In healthy development, the set of preconditions necessary for the elaboration of an oedipal conflict evolve in a stage- and phase-specific manner. Progression in instinctual representation and the formation of mental structures are perfectly matched in meeting developmental needs for advances in differentiation and self-expansion. The fixation point on the projective arm of perception, the grandiose self and ego ideal, and the fixation point on the introjective arm of perception all form in an orderly sequence in concert with the unfolding of the component instincts. This gradual process of structuralizing the personality, during the narcissistic phases of development, prepares the way for a genital consolidation and new level of psychic organization initiated by the formation of an oedipal conflict. There is sufficient stability for the lines of continuity of prohibitive and instinctual experiences to organize into the signaling and regulatory structure of castration anxiety and for the genital instinctual fantasies comprising the oedipal conflict to flourish.

In the developing hysteric, one consequence of the delay in initiating separation and individuation is that these preconditions all transpire over a short time span with excessive overlapping. An oedipal constellation emerges that is inordinately conflicted, which affects the degree of resolution that can be attained, and interferes with work, play and love relationships. There is sufficient structuralization to negotiate the shift from narcissism to object relatedness, but the orderly sequence of events is replaced by compensatory pathological developments.

The consolidation of the component instincts into a genital drive is associated with an increase in instinctual demand, which, in the potential hysteric, affects the organizing structure of castration anxiety. There is an exaggerated need for the prohibitive force of an impinging object because instinctual activity is already potentially overstimulating. The bad impinging qualities of an object that have been represented as devouring during the oral phase and sadistic during the anal phase are only minimally present and have little influence. The impressions of a phallically impinging humiliating object have been predominant and included within self-experience to guard against the expression of voyeuristic impulses. With a genital consolidation, these impinging qualities of an object become more threatening and castrative in nature. They are utilized to expand the process of identification with an aggressor and establish a foundation for the prohibitive function of the superego. The prolonged period of libidinal overinvolvement has also affected the hierarchical organization of narcissistically detemined representations in the id of the dynamic unconscious. Instead of a balanced progression, it is composed of an overabundance of orally derived representations that exert an effect upon the formation of derivatives. Although the selective identifications embodied in the ego ideal have been primarily of bad impinging qualities, the influences of a good object have also been included to offer some degree of self-enhancement. It is by virtue of their presence, in conjunction with the good self-experiences that have been well structuralized within the personality, that the thrust for developmental progression can continue. The narcissistically determined structures forming the necessary preconditions for an oedipal conflict shape its composition and affect the degree of resolution that can be attained. The fixation point on the introjective arm of perception, based upon the good self's bad infantile instinctual qualities, is only relinquished in proportion to the extent of oedipal conflict resolution. The status of this fixation point is the determining factor as to whether hysterical symptoms or hysterical character pathology is manifested.

The Defensive Significance of Hysterical Symptoms and of Hysterical Character Pathology

In healthy development, the fixation point on the introjective arm of perception is maintained for a transient period of time, while the oedipal conflict is organizing new object-related structures at the interior of the personality. The memory traces of infantile instinctual experience provide the necessary stability while these new structures are forming, by limiting the disruptive effects of an influx of new stimuli. The resolution of the oedipal conflict is accomplished through selective identifications, which strengthen the integrative functions in the self-system of representations. Instinctual activity that had previously required defense can be included within good self-experience, and the superego gains dominance as an independent regulatory agency. The resolution of the oedipal conflict is accompanied by an integration of the fixation point on the introjective arm of perception, and new object-related perceptions are registered and represented without defensive interference.

The individual prone to develop hysterical symptoms has formed sufficient structuralization for the thrust of development to attain access to these new object-related experiences, but the oedipal conflict is inadequately resolved, the superego remains polarized in it functions and in opposition to the interests of the ego, and there is only an incomplete and partial integration of the fixation point on the introjective arm of perception. The compromises of symptom formation are required for the introjective arm of perception to be open to new object-related experiences because they are a source of potential overstimulation. Each time the fixation point is relinquished, the threat of overstimulation emerges, and regulation is achieved through the compromises involved in the formation of a symptom. The symptom is designed to manage overstimulation by giving expression to repressed genital instinctual demands disguised by their defensive counterparts, includes a prohibitive superego response and an adaptational compromise with the demands of reality. The symptom will be composed of the body ego experiences most available for symbolic conversion to a disturbance of bodily function. The particular body sensations or bodily functions that are affected are determined by the individual's unique developmental history. A hysterical symptom most often consists of the representation of an orally derived experience of sensory deprivation or libidinal overstimulation that is symbolically elaborated into a distorted bodily sensation, under the influence of poorly regulated phallic and genital instinctual activities. This advanced developmental level of psychopathology occurs upon a foundation in which continuity of experience and cohesiveness are well established, object constancy is secure, and the fixation point on the projective arm of perception is stable and functional, and the fixation point on the introjective arm of perception is partially integrated.

Character pathology functions in opposition to the internalization of new experiences. The individual with hysterical character pathology, faced with a similar set of circumstances, has reacted by establishing a fixed manner of registering perceptions. The phallically determined fixation point on the introjective arm of perception is defensively maintained and is the basis for character attitudes that become solidly entrenched as a response to all stimuli. The oedipal conflict is unresolved and an active force within the personality; the superego remains polarized and in opposition to ego interests; and the fixation points are tenaciously anchored to the phallically determined memory traces of infantile instinctual experience and infantile attachments to an object. The defensive functions of the ego are occupied with maintaining the fixation points and the fixed attitudes that they create and are unavailable to engage in the compromises of symptom formation. Hysterical symptoms are formed upon the foundation of a character structure that is hysterical in its composition. Hysterical character pathology is only manifested when the symptoms are ineffective or when the oedipal conflict has not been sufficiently resolved to even partially integrate the fixation point on the introjective arm of perception.

The effects of hysterical pathology are evidenced in all areas of psychic functioning. The overemphasis upon libidinal stimulation has resulted in an overdeveloped system of self-representations and the underutilized system of object representations. Thinking is dominated by imagery, body sensations, and a reliance on intuitive responses. The delay in forming a fixation point on the projective arm of perception has eventuated in a relatively inactive process of depersonification. The projective mechanisms necessary for intellectual functions are thereby diminished in their effectiveness, and conceptualization and abstract thinking are deficient. The paucity of optimally frustrating experiences has left a reservoir of unrealized potentials, and the hysteric is characteristically an underachiever. There is a preoccupation with the orally influenced, phallically determined meaning of an experience, which is reflected in internal thought, language, and the formation of derivatives. The oedipal conflict is an active threatening internal presence, and the superego functions to direct perceptual attention away from this source of stimulation. Perceptual attention is directed particularly to the defensive structures that have been organized in the self-system of representations to mitigate the state of overstimulation. The process of identification with a humiliating aggressor has effected a reaction formation in the realm of self-experience, which results in a preoccupation with the threat of humiliation. This is designed to prevent the awarness of intense sexual interest in an overstimulating object.

When hysterical symptoms appear in an individual with obsessive character attributes, or conversely obsessive symptoms with hysterical character attributes, it is indicative of fixation points that are highly unstable and not solidly established. Neurotic disorders (hysteric and obsessive) have attained an advanced genital organization, which necessitates the presence of stable fixation points firmly anchored to the memory traces of infantile attachments to an object and to infantile instinctual experience. In healthy development, the fixation point on the introjective arm of perception is integrated and relinquished, and the fixation point on the projective arm of perception is increasingly depersonified and freed of the influence of infantile attachments to an object. A genital character structure then functions to determine the meaning of stimuli without distortion. The character structure of the hysteric and obsessive remains bound to infantile attachments, and when the introjective arm of the perception is stabilized by a defensively maintained fixation point, character pathology is manifested. The stimuli of new experiences are then distorted by the effects of a fixed character attitude. In the hysteric with symptoms, this fixation point is partially integrated and periodically relinquished as a reflection of the thrust for developmental progression. In the obsessive with symptoms, it is relinquished as a reflection of a regressive breakdown in function. Symptoms are only formed when this fixation point is open to new experiences because the defensive functions of the ego that are required in effecting compromises are utilized in maintaining these fixed attitudes. Hysterical symptoms, designed to regulate the influx of new object-related experiences, are formed on the foundation of a hysterical character. Obsessive symptoms, designed to regulate an ineffective repression of instinctual activity, are formed on the foundation of an obsessive character. In narcissistic disorders that have established cohesiveness, a fixation point is maintained on the introjective arm of perception that is not solid and does not effectively prevent the influx of new experience. In combination with the underlying instability of differentiating structures, it leads to a defensive organization that is manifested in differing constellations of pathological compromises. The presence of a mixed picture of neuroticlike symptoms and character traits is associated with a narcissistically organized personality, which will be evident in the overall pattern of psychic functioning.

CHAPTER 3

Hysterical Symptom Formation and Hysterical Character Pathology
Oedipal Determinants

Introduction: Castration Anxiety and the Oedipal Conflict

The limits of instinctual representation within a narcissistically structured personality are reached as the component instincts consolidate into a genital drive. The associative increase in intensity requires the formation of new mental structures to alleviate this potential phobic situation and to enable the continuation of self-expansion and self-differentiation. The stage is set for the genitally determined fantasies of the oedipal situation to exert an organizing influence upon the personality. It is initiated by consolidating the lines of continuity of experience into the structure of castration anxiety, which serves a unique and necessary signaling and regulatory function.

Body ego experiences are registered, represented, and coalesce into discrete entities in accordance with the need for, or inclusion of, defense and form a functional system of self-representations. Good self-experience does not require defense and includes phase-specific instinctual gratification, the activity of autonomous ego functions, and the background object of primary identification (Grotstein, 1981; Mendelsohn, 1985). Bad self-experience involves defense and includes instinctual overstimulation, sensory deprivations, and reactions to impingement. Although present as separate entities, a connection exists in the realm of instinctual experience because instinctual activity is on a continuum of intensity that gradually instigates a defensive response. A functional system of object representations is formed from the object-impression counterparts that are registered and also that coalesce into discrete entities. The impressions of a good object do not elicit defense and include the qualities of optimal gratification, optimal frustration, and of a transitional object. The impressions of a bad object elicit defense and include the qualities of instinctual over-stimulation, deprivation, and impingement. These are also present as separate entities but maintain a connection in the realm of the restraining influences of an object. Optimal frustration, which is represented as an aspect of a good object, gradually shades into prohibitions and the impingements of bad object. It is the recognition of these lines of continuity of experience that is at the foundation of the fixation points, and their consolidation forms the structure of castration anxiety.

Castration anxiety is represented as an instinctual self in contact with a prohibitive object. At its extreme, instinctual intensity is heightened, and the prohibitive qualities of the object are castrative in nature. At its mildest, instinctual activity is contained, and the object offers gentle restraint. It reflects the underlying union of both good and bad qualities in the self and object and is a manifestation of its regulatory function, as any increase in instinctual activity mobilizes more forceful prohibitions. This feature of combining all aspects of mental representation enables the capacity to signal the need for additional defense, which is an essential condition for the oedipal fantasies to fully flourish.

The oedipal situation refers to the representation of genital instinctual self-experience and a genital instinctual object's influence and the fantasies that are elaborated from them. It has conscious, preconscious, and unconscious components, is included within good and bad self-experiences, and involves the good and bad impressions of an object. The oedipal conflict refers to those aspects of the oedipal situation, requiring or eliciting defense, that are elaborated into fantasies expressive of unconscious wishes. These fantasies exert an organizing influence by providing the linkages, structuralized at the interior, that establish the capacity to represent increasing quantities of instinctual demand from an object-related perspective. The demands of biophysiology are on a continuum of intensity that has been represented with differing qualities. A dimension not requiring defense is included within good self-experience as phase-specific instinctual gratifications; a dimension attaining overstimulating qualities is included within self-experience with the aid of defense and is represented as a facet of the bad self, and a dimension possesses an intensity that cannot be included within self-experience but leaves an impression having the independent qualities of an overstimulating instinctual object. This is the portal of entry of instinctual demand, represented as a bad instinctual object, which has necessitated the greatest degree of defensive opposition during the narcissistic phases of development. It has stood as an obstacle to sustaining a continuous uninterrupted flow of instinctual demand, moving toward representation within the realm of self-experience, where there is access to the integrative functions of the ego. The continuum of biophysiological demand has a further unseen, unperceivable dimension, which has had a traumatic impact on the narcissistically structured personality. This dimension has to be defensively excluded from representation until the genital fantasies of the oedipal conflict establish a structured pathway that enables the perception of unseen stimuli.

The representation of a bad genital instinctual object is elaborated into a primal scene fantasy, which captures the essence of the unseen dimension of instinctual demand. It is the fantasy of an unseen object, hidden but perceived and responded to as ominous, mysterious, and instinctually overstimulating. This fantasy is linked to the representation of self-experiences of genital overstimulation, which reflects the libidinal search for an object. The union is structured to form a pathway by which instinctual demand gains continuous access into the self-system of representations. Instinctual activity that previously was defensively excluded from representation can now be included, and the initial step necessary for integration, sublimation, and secondary autonomy has been negotiated. In the primal scene fantasy, the self is represented as observing an unseen genital sexual object and becoming overstimulated. It both expresses and manifests the pathway of instinctual integration, reflects the capacity to perceive the unseen dimensions of biophysiologic demand, and insures cohesiveness at the interior.

The representation of bad genital instinctual self-experience is elaborated into an incestuous fantasy, which embodies forbidden, prohibitive qualities reflecting the mobilization of defense. These incestuous fantasies are linked to the representation of a bad instinctual object, uniting the self- and object systems in a defensive and regulatory direction. The union is structured to establish a new object-related boundary for the id of the dynamic unconscious. The boundaries that define the conscious and preconscious systems incorporate focused areas of perceptual activity, but the boundary of the unconscious system must be devoid of perceptual functions. However, it must be flexible enough to evoke the formation of derivatives and maintain continuity of experience within the personality.

This bilateral structural union is formed during the oedipal period, unites the self- and object systems of representation in two opposing directions, establishes the foundation for object-related perceptions, and insures cohesiveness at the interior. The representations of a bad genital instinctual object and of bad genital instinctual self-experience are structurally united to form a pathway of instinctual integration, manifested by primal scene fantasies, and a new boundary for the id of the dynamic unconscious, manifested by incestuous fantasies. In a clinical situation, the expression of incestuous fantasies is accompanied by the mobilization of defense associated with the structure maintaining a boundary for the unconscious system. The expression of primal scene fantasies is indicative of a movement toward further integration and is accompanied by self-expansion. Primal scene fantasies are characterized by the presence of instinctual overstimulation with the object remaining unseen. It is not an explicit sexual scene involving objects that are perceived. Incestuous fantasies involve explicit sexual scenes with forbidden primary infantile objects or their derivatives.

The increased capacity for instinctual representation provides the impetus and motivation for resolution of the oedipal conflict through selective identifications. Influences of an object are included within self-experience to strengthen adaptive and integrative functions; this enables the final step in the pathway of instinctual integration to be negotiated. Instinctual experience that had previously required defense can be represented as a facet of good self-experience and has attained secondary autonomy. Concomitantly, the superego consolidates as an independently functioning agency, and its varied functions are harmoniously interrelated with the interests of the ego. The fixation points are gradually freed of their tenacious attachment to the representations of infantile objects and narcissistic instinctual experiences, to facilitate self-enhancement through object-related experiences. The change in the fixation points involves a process of depersonification on the projective arm of perception and of integration on the introjective arm of perception. In the hysteric, pathological effects are exhibited in all areas of development pertaining to the emergence and resolution of the oedipal conflict.

An individual displaying hysterical pathology has successfully negotiated separation and individuation and has developed sufficient structuralization of the personality for the oedipal conflict to form. A foundation for object-related experiences has been established, although they operate as a source of potential trauma rather than of enhancement. A partial resolution of an inordinately conflicted oedipal constellation may be achieved, but it necessitates the formation of symptoms as a regulatory measure. The events of early development have a continuing effect upon the progressive steps of later development, which is reflected in the mental structures that have formed in preparation for the shift from narcissism to object relatedness. The libidinal overinvolvement of the oral phase has left an overabundance of object impressions dominated by the influence of the nurturing maternal figure, which has an effect on the functioning of the superego. The delay in separation and individuation also has an effect upon the structural composition of castration anxiety and shapes the particular configuration of oedipal fantasies. The intensity of the oedipal conflict is exaggerated by the nature of the attachment to the maternal figure.

The Influence of Early Development upon the Structure of Castration Anxiety and the Oedipal Conflict

In healthy development, the recognition of a separate good object's influence takes place during the anal phase when experiences of mastery and control are in the ascendency. A fixation point is established on the projective arm of perception, based upon the good object's bad anal qualities, which anchors object constancy and sets the stage for the formation of mental structures that further unite and differentiate the self- and object systems of representation. These structures, the grandiose self and ego ideal, create the boundaries within which the superego consolidates into an independently functioning agency. The grandiose self is constructed with the anally determined fantasies of an object's omnipotence, which provides just the right balance for the vulnerability associated with the recognition of separateness. The ego ideal is constructed with just the right phallically determined influences of an object that strengthen integrative and adaptive functions. Stage and phase specificities have reference to this match of available mental representations, consonant with a developmental need, for progress in self-expansion to continue. When that synchronized pattern is disturbed, compensatory responses are instigated creating distortions in the movement toward developmental advancement.

In the developing hysteric, formation of a fixation point on the projective arm of perception is delayed until the phallic phase, and object constancy is anchored by a good object's bad humiliating qualities. Instinctual expansion has taken place without the orderly sequence of stage and phase specificity, which results in the grandiose self and ego ideal being structured to establish cohesiveness without effective restraints for instinctual activity. The need for identifications with an aggressor is exaggerated, and a phallically determined prohibitive response at this stage of psychic organization is limited in its effectiveness. When development proceeds in accord with stage and phase specificity, there may also be a need for identifications with an aggressor. However, this occurs at moments of stress, is transient, and the available influences of an object are very effective in providing restraint and regulation. The grandiose self and ego ideal of the hysteric form at a time when the developmental need is for enhancement of phallic exhibitionism. The heightened necessity for including the humiliating influences of a phallically derived bad impinging object, within self-experience, interferes with the phase-specific needs of phallic instinctual activity.

The optimally gratifying impressions of a phallically determined good object are represented as an object's reflecting and admiring the phallic exhibitionistic qualities of self-experience. Optimally frustrating impressions are represented as offering restraint by evoking functions that instigate control from within. The hysteric has a deficiency in these optimally frustrating influences, and the mental structures that maintain differentiation and regulation are not stage and phase specific and have formed rapidly. The consolidation of the component instincts into a genital drive, which in health is an impetus to integrative functions, leads to a greater degree of instability and an inordinate need for defense.

In the orderly sequence of healthy development, each new structure that forms exerts a stabilizing effect upon the succeeding steps. The formation of fixation points, the grandiose self and ego ideal, and the consolidation of the lines of continuity of experience into the structure of castration anxiety lay a solid foundation for the unfolding of the oedipal situation. The oedipal conflict then functions as a psychic organizer, forming a new boundary for the id of the dynamic unconscious, a new structured and continuous pathway of instinctual integration, and facilitating the formation of defensive unions needed for regulation. Each step accomplishes a developmental task with the formation of mental structures particularly suited to phase-specific needs. Each advancement offers an opportunity to more effectively integrate that which was difficult in the preceding steps. Each new evolution incorporates the preceding structures into an expanded level of psychic organization. In this intermeshing of stage- and phase-specific tasks, there is a harmonious interplay of forces. Whenever an element is not in harmony, it affects each succeeding step. In the hysteric, the nature of early experience has been such that the most significant tasks of psychic structuralization can be negotiated. However, developmental sequences are out of synchrony with stage and phase specificity, and though the compensatory effects create difficulty, they do not interfere with the thrust for progression until the demands of resolving the oedipal conflict are reached.

Definable categories of pathology are a product of excessive deficiencies, traumatic impingements, or both. The hysteric has had a combination of libidinal experiences that were overstimulating to the point of impingement and an insufficiency of those optimally frustrating influences that are evocative to autonomous functioning. The emphasis upon orality is reflected in the abundance of orally determined representations of self-experience and of an object's influence that ultimately comprise the id of the dynamic unconscious, that are included in the expression of derivatives, and that are utilized in the formation of symptomatic compromises. The anal phase is both short lasting and affected by an extension of the libidinal overinvolvement of the oral period. Anality is not a difficult or conflictual period, nor is it a differentiating one. The developing sense of autonomy, control, and mastery is not sufficiently amplified, which contributes to the already existing deficit in the use of potential functions. Nontraumatic qualities of impingement and deprivation, in balanced proportions, play an essential role in fostering defensive functions, adaptive capacities, and in furthering self-differentiation. These bad qualities are not properly balanced so that the regulatory forces in the personality are unable to gradually diminish the need for external regulation.

The formation of a fixation point on the introjective arm of perception offers enough stability for castration anxiety to consolidate as a signaling and regulatory structure. However, it is unduly prohibitive because the restraints that evolve gradually through stage and phase specificity are largely unavailable. Castration anxiety assumes an enormous burden as the most effective regulatory influence and enables the genital fantasies of the oedipal conflict to structuralize the shift from narcissism to object relatedness. The capacity for representing the unseen dimension of biophysiological demand and for perceiving the independent qualities of an object is established but is potentially traumatic. The diminution in activity of autonomous ego functions and the overdevelopment of sensory deprivations match the compensatory need to form defensive unions designed to adapt to phallic and genital overstimulation. The hysteric with symptoms has progressed sufficiently to achieve a partial resolution of the oedipal conflict and with it a periodic relinquishing of the fixation point on the introjective arm of perception. The resulting threat of overstimulation is managed by the compromises effected in the symptom.

The Oedipal Conflict in Hysteria

Prior to the elaboration of an oedipal conflict, the line of continuity of instinctual experience is readily interrupted. Phase-specific instinctual gratification is represented within good self-experience, shades into bad self-experience as the intensity mounts and defenses are instituted, and maintains a tenuous connection to the portal of entry of instinctual demand represented as a bad instinctual object. The oedipal conflict structures that connection by organizing a pathway of instinctual integration and a new boundary for the unconscious system. Primal scene fantasies reflect an instinctual movement toward integration, which, in the hysteric, is fraught with danger and must be vigorously defended against. A solid, well-structured pathway of instinctual integration has formed but is experienced as a threat. Incestuous fantasies reflect the activity of the structured boundary for the unconscious system, which is associated with a heightening of defensive responses and, in the hysteric, is overdeveloped. The interrelationship of these structures is indicative of the degree of conflict engendered by the oedipal fantasies. In health, primal scene fantasies predominate, whereas in hysteria, incestuous fantasies are most prevalent.

The effects of libidinal overinvolvement during the earlier phases of development have a powerful impact upon the oedipal situation. In the female, the maternal figure is maintained as a genital instinctual object for an inordinate period of time that exaggerates the tenacity of a negative oedipal attachment. The developmental task of displacing genital interest to the father is fraught with the danger of overstimulation and instigates strong defensive opposition. The impressions of a male object's influences, which have been represented in the shadow of the primary object, lend themselves to being registered with the qualities of the unseen aspect of instinctual demand. The male is then perceived as an instinctual presence, represented as a bad seductive overstimulating genital sexual object, and must be actively defended against.

In the male, the libidinal overinvolvement with the primary object intensifies the genital instinctual attachment, and an extremely powerful prohibitive force is required for it to be effectively repressed. The impressions of a male object's influence, represented in the shadow of the dominant primary maternal object, are relatively sparse and registered with the qualities of a genitally impinging object. The male figure is then perceived as a castrative threat. A negative oedipal position offers no solution to the male hysteric because it would require a denial of the penis as the symbolic organ of connection to an object. The hysteric's emphasis upon phallic experience has fostered a narcissistic overevaluation of the penis. Conversion symptoms may involve impotence or inhibition of genital discharge as a response to the threat of castration, but the penis is too highly valued to be defensively relinquished. In addition, the instinctual attachment to the female is too strong a bond to be defensively detached.

When the fixation point on the introjective arm of perception has attained some degree of integration and is open to receive new experiences, the resulting stimuli evoke the activity of the representation of a bad instinctual object. This triggers the compromises expressed in hysterical conversion symptoms and allows the introjective arm of perception to remain open. When there is an insufficient integration of instinctual demand and the fixation point on the introjective arm of perception is defensively maintained, the fixed phallically determined attitudes of hysterical character pathology are manifested.

The Defensive Organization in the Hysteric

During the course of healthy development, castration anxiety is consolidated as a structure in a stage- and phase-specific manner, is a modulated effective regulator of instinctual activity, and signals for the institution of defensive responses that faciliate a continuous movement toward instinctual integration. In hysteria, the structure of castration anxiety is consolidated under stress, is a poor regulator of instinctual activity, and signals for the institution of defensive responses that act in opposition to continuing integration. The emerging genital fantasies of the oedipal conflict are affected by this exaggerated need for defense.

The initial stages of repression proper occur with a superego that is polarized in its functions. Perceptual attention is directed away from the source of a threatening stimulus and toward that which is least threatening. With the resolution of the oedipal conflict, the self-system of representations is strengthened through selective identifications, the superego functions are unified, and perceptual attention can be directed at the source of a stimulus. The hysteric has not achieved a resolution of the oedipal conflict, the superego remains polarized in its functions, and perceptual attention continues to be directed away from a source of stimulation. Frustration is a response reflecting the presence of defensive opposition to instinctual discharge, is indicative of an emerging state of overstimulation, and involves much sensory activity. Deprivation is a response reflecting an absence of sensory stimulation, is elaborated into a fantasy of emptiness, and serves well as a defense against overstimulation. With the increase in instinctual demand associated with an oedipal conflict, perceptual attention is directed to the representations of sensory deprivation that are linked to the impressions of a depriving object through the fantasy of emptiness. This defensive union ameliorates the potentially traumatic effects of overstimulation.

The impinging impressions of an object are shaped by the instinctual impact of biophysiological demands, so that they are represented in accordance with the advancing stages of psychosexual development. During the oral phase, they are incorporative; with anality, they are sadistic; and, as the phallic and genital phases predominate, they are humiliating and castrative in nature. In healthy development, there is a balanced progression, which provides the prohibitive influences of an object that are necessary for transient identifications with an aggressor at moments of stress or overstimulation. The hysteric has established reaction formations by including the hypertrophied influences of a humiliating phallic object within self-experience, in order to control poorly regulated voyeuristic impulses. These are at the foundation of the hysteric's character structure and reenforce the fixed attitudes expressive of pathology.

The underemphasis upon autonomous functioning and the excessive degree of sensory deprivation in other than instinctual modalities result in the availability of body ego experiences of deprivation and absence of function, which are utilized in the formation of conversion symptoms. The emphasis upon oral and phallic instinctual experience creates the readiness for libidinization of these conversion reactions and aids in instinctual regulation. Every stimulus, whether it emanates from the internal or external world, has the potential for becoming overstimulating. Primal scene fantasies are especially threatening and mobilize a pathological response manifested in the formation of hysterical symptoms or in the fixed attitudes of hysterical character pathology. Incestuous fantasies and their derivatives are overdeveloped as an expression of this defensive orientation to instinctual demand.

The Status and Significance of Object-Related Perceptions in the Hysteric

In healthy development, the oedipal conflict functions as a psychic organizer by structuring an object-related orientation to the stimuli of the internal and external worlds. This enables the capacity to perceive an external object as having independent objects of its own and to register the unseen dimension of biophysiological demands. The mental structures at the foundation of these object-related perceptions ensure cohesiveness at the interior of the personality and facilitate a continuous flow of instinctual activity from its portal of entry at the interior to attaining secondary autonomy at the periphery. This new structured pathway of instinctual integration, along with a newly formed regulatory boundary for the unconscious system, serves as a motivating force for the resolution of the oedipal conflict through selective identifications. Integrative functions are strengthened, instinctual activities that had previously required defense can be included within good self-experience, the fixation point on the introjective arm of perception is relinquished, and a conflict-free system of functions assumes increasing dominance. Concomitantly, the superego's varied functions are unified and operate in harmony with the interests of the ego. Continuity of experience is secure, and repression proper no longer requires perceptual attention to be directed away from a source of stimulation.

The hysteric has established the capacity for object-related perceptions, but that developmental step is poorly negotiated and fraught with anxiety. Object-related experiences are a potential source of trauma, rather than enhancement, and instigate an inordinate defensive response. The oedipal conflict is at best only partially resolved, and the particular manifestations of pathology depend upon the degree of resolution. The varied functions of the superego remain polarized and in opposition to the interests of the ego. Repression proper continues to operate by directing perceptual attention away from the source of a stimulus and toward that which is least threatening.

The fixation point on the introjective arm of perception, which was formed to provide the necessary stability for the oedipal conflict to elaborate, is either defensively maintained or if relinquished is in a state of readiness to be reestablished. To the extent that the oedipal conflict is resolved, the memory traces of infantile instinctual experience forming the fixation point are integrated. This allows new object-related experiences to be registered with the support and regulation of hysterical conversion symptoms because the compromises involved in a symptom are designed to manage the resulting state of overstimulation. Orally influenced body ego experiences of sensory deprivation and unrealized potentials are utilized to symbollically express phallic and genital instinctual activities. The symptom embodies the ego's defensive opposition, the superego's prohibitive response, and an adaptive component designed to attain reenforcement from external objects. Thus, in the presence of a symptom, the introjective arm of perception can remain open to register new object-related experiences.

When a symptom is ineffective in regulating instinctual activity or when there has been an insufficient degree of resolution of the oedipal conflict, the introjective arm of perception remains fixated by the memory traces of infantile phallic instinctual experience. All stimuli are given a phallically determined meaning, and hysterical character pathology is manifested. *Character structure* has reference to the particular composition of the mental structures that function as a background for registering perceptions and for determining adaptive responses to the stimuli of the inner and outer world. *Character pathology* refers to the manner in which perceptions are distorted by the influence of that structural foundation. *Hysterical symptoms* are embedded in a hysterical character structure and reflect the attempt to further the thrust for continuing self-expansion. Hysterical character pathology is in evidence when distortions are created and obviates against developmental progression.

The Effects of Hysteric Development upon Thinking, Perception, and Adaptation

The delay in recognition of the good object's bad qualities tends to foster a denial of separateness, to blur the sense of differentiation, and to extend the period of dependence on an external object for the maintenance of self-esteem. Inevitable narcissistic injuries have an excessive impact, and self-regulatory functions are underdeveloped. The hysteric individual sustains the impression of being surrounded by the libidinal overinvolvement of an object, which reinforces an attitude of lack of recognition of unpleasant aspects of the external world.

Thinking is dominated by imagery, and there is a diminished capacity to utilize intellectual processes or to think in abstract terms. The fixation point on the projective arm of perception, which functions to anchor object constancy and support projective mechanisms, is not sufficiently depersonified. One consequence is in a style of thinking and language that reflects the hypertrophy of instinctual body ego experiences and their representation. Conceptualizations and abstract thought are inhibited, and intuitive, feeling responses are overemphasized. Perceptions are strongly affected by these feeling reactions; this creates both an exquisite sensitivity and an exquisite insensitivity to the significance of an experience. When the introjective arm of perception is open to register new object-related experiences, without the distorting effects of a fixation point, the hysteric can accurately determine the qualities present in an interaction. When the fixation point is defensively maintained, this ability to discriminate is lost.

The conflict-free sphere is organized into a system of autonomous ego functions at the point of perceptual contact with the external world. In healthy development, instinctual demands traverse a structured pathway of integration, ultimately attaining secondary autonomy and forming a boundary for this conflict-free sector of the personality. In the hysteric, instinctual demands attaining secondary autonomy are extremely sparse, and the conflict-free sphere is poorly defined as a system of functions. Although object constancy, cohesiveness, and continuity of experience have been established, and in some a partial resolution of the oedipal conflict, adaptive responses continue to be determined by the representations of infantile experience.

Some Implications for Treatment

The psychic organization of the hysteric is cohesive, object related, and characterized by a readiness for phallic and genital instinctual ovestimulation. Pathological defenses are manifested in response to the stimuli of the internal and external worlds, on the background of an active and unresolved oedipal conflict. When the stimuli of external interactions possess qualities that are impinging, depriving, or overstimulating, the defensive response is instigated by the activity of unconscious perceptions, and their derivatives will express these pathological qualities. In the presence of an unconsciously empathic environment, which does not elicit a pathological adaptive response, the source of stimulation emanates primarily from the internal world. Defenses are then initiated by the activity of primal scene and incestuous fantasies.

The therapeutic environment must contain the combined qualities of a good object and be free of surprises that are a potential source of overstimulation. These conditions are evocative of healthy modes of interaction, and the character of the hysteric will emerge in bold relief. The therapist's management of a familiar, contained framework with well-defined boundaries and ground rules, within which interpretations of unconscious strivings are offered, is optimally gratifying to the thrust for growth and self-expansion. Abstaining from participating in the reinforcement of pathological defenses serves to amplify the underdeveloped autonomous ego functions and is optimally frustrating. The encouragement of a freely associative process that faciliates the expression of transference wishes has the qualities of a transitional object. The hysteric who begins treatment, displaying symptoms, has achieved a partial resolution of the oedipal conflict and will recreate a new edition in the transference relationship without the necessity of the compromises involved in a symptom. When the environment is overstimulating, symptoms will emerge, and if they are ineffective in their regulatory function, the fixed attitudes of hysterical character pathology will result. An individual with hysterical symptoms giving evidence of character pathology may be responding to overstimulating qualities in an interaction, and the source may be the behavior of the therapist.

Hysterical character pathology is manifested in a fixed way of perceiving the stimuli of an interaction and presents a different therapeutic need. Interpretive words may have very little impact on the manner in which experience is determined. The memory traces of infantile attachments to an object and of infantile instinctual experiences that comprise the fixation points and the differentiating structures of the grandiose self and ego ideal have maintained their original narcissistically determined qualities. The infantile representations must be replaced to some degree, for perception to gain a measure of independence from their influence.

The grandiose self is based upon a narcissistic attachment in which phallic exhibitionism is enhanced by the fantasized admiration of an object. The conscious experience of an interaction is influenced by this perception. Simultaneously, the interaction is evocative to more deeply preconscious and unconscious representations of instinctual activities. These mobilize the prohibitive influences of a humiliating and castrating object. Reverberating with the conscious experience of the therapist as an optimally gratifying phallic audience is the preconscious experience of a potential humiliator and/or castrator and the unconscious experience of a genital instinctual object. The hysteric, in expressing poorly regulated exhibitionistic activities, is often described as seductive, flamboyant, or histrionic. Interpretations that are directed to these surface qualities of what appears to be a seductive attitude are readily perceived as humiliating. They do not consider the underlying preconscious and unconscious meanings and may reflect the therapist's defensiveness. Interventions that are offered from a defensive posture reenforce a patient's character pathology and recreate the conditions in which it had formed.

The ego ideal is based upon a narcissistic attachment, in which admired influences of an object are included within self-experience to aid in the regulation of phallic instinctual activity. The influence of this structure is predominant in determining adaptive responses and is most accessible to the effects of a therapeutic interaction, particularly in the early phases. Object impressions of the interaction can then become available to replace the original infantile representations, enabling a degree of independence from their influence. Optimally frustrating qualities are especially significant in strengthening adaptive capacities and enhancing integrative functions. It is only when the infantile attachments and infantile experiences at the foundation of the fixation points are exposed to view that the oedipal fantasies can be fully expressed in the transference relationship.

Depression in the Hysteric

There are as many differing forms and experiences of depression as there are differing ways of perceiving the inner and outer worlds. Depression as a diagnostic category, having a unique set of dynamics, does not fit with its varied manifestations. The original formulation of the dynamics of depression were in relation to melancholia and were instrumental in leading to the structural hypothesis and a clearer understanding of the superego. The dynamics delineated in the melancholic were applied to all depressions and not returned to for revision. Depression is a phenomenum associated with each diagnostic category, in which the individual is responding to an internal loss. The particular form it takes is dependent upon the nature of the loss and the way it is perceived. Depression conceptualized in this way is not a specific diagnostic entity with a unique set of dynamics and a particular structural composition but is an internal loss expressed in accordance with the personality organization of a given diagnostic category. Individuals with hysterical lines of development experience depression in a similar way because the nature of the internal loss and the response to it are alike. Depression in obsessional, phobic, borderline, and schizophrenic forms of pathologies possess differences, which are the result of variances in the specific nature of the internal loss and in the way it is perceived and adapted to. Reactions to the loss of an external object are not an expression of depression, unless it is evocative of an internal loss.

The hysteric has developed the capacity for recognizing that an external object has unseen objects of its own and an independent sexual existence. This ability to perceive the effects of unseen objects is reflected in the primal scene fantasies that enable the representation of the unseen dimension on the continuum of biophysiological demand and that are structuralized to form a pathway of instinctual integration. The hysteric, under the influence of defensive responses to instinctual overstimulation, does not allow a continuous influx of instinctual activity along this pathway, and it is inaccessible to the integrative functions of the ego.

Two major structures are formed during the oedipal period to unite the self- and object representational systems at the interior. One forms a new boundary for the unconscious system, and one establishes a structured pathway of integration that insures a continuous flow of instinctual activity. In addition, the representations of deprivation and impingement are united with their object-impression counterparts to serve a defensive function. The superego, in its early stages of organization, regulates repression by directing perceptual attention away from a threatening source of stimulation. Perceptual attention is then directed to these defensive unions when the conflict engendered by the primal scene fantasies is inordinate. At these moments, there is a loss of direct contact with the representations of an overstimulating instinctual object. The depression of the hysteric is a response to this loss and is expressed in a preoccupation with deprivation and impingement. The derivatives of an overstimulating instinctual object are repressed, as the fantasies of emptiness and reactions to impingement occupy perceptual attention.

The internal loss is related to the effects of having attained sufficient structuralization to respond to the continuing thrust for developmental progression. The differences between the individual with symptoms and with character pathology depend upon the degree of oedipal conflict resolution, the degree to which the fixation point on the introjective arm of perception has been integrated, and the degree to which new object-related experiences can be registered. In the presence of character pathology, this depression is constantly in the background, whereas with symptom formation it is episodic.

CHAPTER 4

Hysterical Symptom Formation and Hysterical Character Pathology
Clinical Material

Clinical Material

A, a very thin 22-year-old unmarried woman, was in great distress. Her symptom of vomiting prevented her from many desired activities. She could never go out to eat because she feared she might vomit and be extremely humiliated. On the occasions that she went out, she was preoccupied with her fear of being humiliated. She also felt she was not living up to her capacities. She worked as a secretary, had avoided further eduction, and regretted it. In her work situation, she felt unhappy and was plagued by a silent attachment to the man for whom she worked. She was powerfully affected by feelings of jealousy in response to hearing any talk of his family. She was terrified of heterosexual relationships, was frequently sought out by men her age, and always avoided this contact.

A became engaged in a psychoanalytic process and spent the first months talking relatively freely of her life, of her experiences in growing up, and of her wishes and aspirations. Verbalizations by the therapist were felt by her as infantilizing or as an interference. A comment or question by the therapist would instigate a dream in which some obstacle interfered with her progress, and she appeared most comfortable in the therapist's silence. Her father had been in service the first 3 years of her life, and two siblings were born at 1 and 3 years after his return. She spoke of her mother with much contempt, stressing her subjugation to her husband and lack of aspirations for herself. She implicitly and derivatively communicated an intense feeling of closeness and uneasiness as to its erotic significance. She was close to female companions and fearful of males. She adhered to a perception of the therapist as strictly a listening and helping figure.

A then had a series of openly incestuous dreams in which she was involved in a sexual interaction with her father. Her attitude in reporting the dreams was one of mild curiosity and puzzlement as to how she could have such inner experiences. The following session occurred immediately afterwards. *A* entered, lay on the couch, and began to feel an intense itching on her inner thigh. She spoke of it with great embarrassment and hesitation. She wanted to scratch but felt immobilized in the therapist's presence. The sensation built in intensity until she had to scratch it. As she did, she recalled how little she knew of sexual matters. She recalled the shock of her first menstrual period. It was not the blood but the realization of an opening in her body that she had no idea existed. As *A* talked, she became restless and, for the first time, expressed an intense desire for the therapist to talk. Previously, the therapist's words were unwanted. The wish to hear the therapist's words mounted, "Why won't you talk?" She went on to hesitantly express her fear that the therapist thought she was masturbating. She knew this had never been a part of her life. She has heard others speak of it, but in no way had she engaged in such a practice. She then recalled being teased as a child for going to the bathroom so frequently. She also remembered her almost driven efforts to wipe herself and noticed a similarity to the itching sensation. The request for the therapist's words escalated to a demand. 'Won't you talk!" The therapist stated that as she itched, she also felt an intense longing for the therapist to bring something to her to relieve her itch. It looked as though those two sensations were connected. *A* began to giggle and to cry. A silly joke she had heard when she was small came to mind. She wanted to laugh even though what it meant did not seem funny. "I feel like I'm the hot dog bun and you are the hot dog." *A* became silent and thought of the feeling in her throat that instigated an episode of vomiting. It was an itching sensation. When she scratched the inside of her thigh, she thought of her throat and became aware of sensations in her genitals. *A* then remembered that the day before the dreams she had left her gloves in the therapist's office. She had returned to get them, the door was closed, and she knew the therapist was with someone. She felt terrified, quickly turned and left, and tried to put it out of her mind.

B, an 8-year-old girl, entered psychotherapy following her mother's contact with school. The mother had ben informed that *B* was an underachiever. She daydreamed and ignored any situation that demanded effort and concentration. The school had done psychological testing, and the examiner had commented that this was the most deprived child she had ever seen. This was a shock to the mother who felt she had provided *B* with everything she needed.

B was eager to come to her sessions and to express her inner trouble. She felt constantly frustrated, bored, and suffered from what she called "growing pains." She felt pains in her body everywhere. They felt like something was trapped and trying to grow. In the early months, she had many and varied pains in her ankles, fingers, stomach, and so forth. She became extremely irritable and upset with the therapist. She had the powerful sense that the therapist did not believe her and was laughing at her inside. Furthermore, it made no difference what the therapist would say or do or how he would respond. She just knew this was how he felt. Nothing could alter that feeling, and it was terribly upsetting to her. The therapist responded by stating that in a way *B* was right and that he did not believe her. He also felt that *B* did not believe the therapist would be able to hear the way in which her body was talking to her. She seemed to fear that the therapist could not read her body's language and that she would therefore remain trapped. *B* immediately began to talk about exploring caves, forests, bushes, and jungles. She was filled with fantasies of the thrill and danger in these explorations. The therapist said he thought her mind was occupied with exploring these places because she wanted the therapist to help her talk about exploring her body and its inner parts. *B* paused, silently went to the couch, and began to masturbate. She talked softly about the therapist's words giving her permission to do what she had wanted to do ever since she began to see him. She felt blocked in talking and had always known that the only way she could talk was to masturbate. The experience of rubbing herself removed the blocks, and her words came easily. She talked about a young, wild cousin and their sexual exploratory games. She recalled having seen a guard at a tollbooth who frightened her and who reminded her of this cousin. She spoke of her overinvolvement with her mother. She wanted to be free of her, yet felt she could not survive without her. The mother and father were divorced when the patient was 2 years old. *B* had periodic visits with her father; these were both exciting and frightening. When with her father, she felt pulled to return to the mother. When she was back with her mother, she experienced an excited wish to return to her father.

C, a 35-year-old divorced woman, entered psychotherapy concerned about moving from one troubled and conflicted love affair to another. She felt driven toward intense relationships that always ended in rejection and recognized she was inciting the trouble. She was anxious about her feeling of attraction to women and made efforts to deny it. In addition, she felt incomplete in her functioning at work.

In the early hours, *C* spoke at length of her anxiety about the use of the couch, which fluctuated with a recognition that it would be best for her. She noticed that she was drawn to searching for the therapist's responses and reactions in order to gain an inner feeling of security and could see this was preventing her from thinking and talking about inner feelings. She then decided to use the couch, and the following session occurred shortly afterward.

C entered the office in a braless revealing T-shirt and was seemingly unaware that her body movements on the couch exposed her breasts to the therapist. The therapist was silently recalling early hours in which *C* had described her previous therapeutic contacts. She was totally offended and frightened by interpretive comments concerning her ''seductive'' behavior. The fact that it was mentioned before she noticed or felt it meant to her that there was something in the other person that was frightened of her or would be seductive to her. She reacted by leaving, never to return. The therapist watched what appeared to be a seductive scene, silently. *C* began to talk about situations in which people saw something, said nothing about it, and as a consequence were untrustable. She became uneasy, irritable, concerned that her words could be heard in the waiting room, and wondered aloud if the room was properly soundproofed. The therapist stated that when he was silent and said nothing about her body's communications to himself or of his awareness of what *C* was displaying, he gave her reason to distrust his motives. *C* reacted by becoming totally humiliated. She felt out on a limb and exposed. She had not realized what she had done. She had awakened late, and, in her rush to get to the session, she had dressed quickly with no thought as to her appearance. She had no place to hide. She fell silent and anxiously spoke of her awareness of the sound of the therapist's breathing. She thought he was sexually aroused and masturbating and then was flooded with memories of her father when she was 7 and 8 years old. He had been a schoolteacher out of work, fired for child molestation. He was at home while her mother worked. *C* came home from school, her father was on the couch, he then held her, became sexually aroused, and masturbated.

Discussion

Hysterical pathology is characterized by an overemphasis upon instinctual experiences with oral and phallic-genital qualities. This was evident in *A*'s symptom of vomiting, which was instigated by an itching sensation having a genitally determined meaning. *B* and *C* frequently expressed instinctual derivatives that were orally influenced and phallically determined. *C* often felt compelled to eat before her sessions, yet felt hungry and fantasied the therapist's having "food hidden in your drawers." *B* had many associations to eating when genitally aroused.

Object constancy, cohesiveness, and continuity of experience were well established in all three patients, and the autonomous ego functions were underdeveloped. *A* was a secretary with a strong inner sense of unrealized potentials; *B* was an "underachiever"; and *C* was unable to utilize her talents and skills due to conflict. All three responded to the optimally frustrating qualities of the therapeutic interaction by amplifying their existing functional abilities.

The experiences of sensory deprivation and reactions to impingement were overdeveloped and used defensively to manage phallic and genital overstimulation. *A* attempted to focus attention upon the therapist's silence and her feeling of deprivation when genital sensations were mounting in intensity. *B* felt impinged upon by a perception of the therapist as a humiliator, which distracted her from being overstimulated. *C* was preoccupied with the humiliation of exposure in response to the phallic and genital experiences that were moving toward expression.

Genital primal scene fantasies are structurally linked to self-experiences of genital overstimulation, during the oedipal period, to form a pathway of instinctual integration. Concomitantly incestuous fantasies are structurally linked to the impressions of an overstimulating genital instinctual object to form a new boundary for the unconscious system. These new object-related structures enable the representation of the unseen dimension of biophysiologic demand and the recognition that an external object has independent objects of its own. Primal scene fantasies are associated with the ascendency of integrative functions, and incestuous fantasies are associated with a heightening of defensive activity. When properly balanced, a continuous, uninterrupted flow of instinctual demand is ensured. In the hysteric, these genitally determined oedipal constellations engender an inordinate degree of conflict; incestuous fantasies are hypertrophied, and primal scene fantasies are a source of potential trauma. This was most noticeable in *A*. She presented openly incestuous dreams with an attitude of mild puzzlement and with no idea as to their source. The effectiveness of repression and predominance of defensive responses was clearly in evidence. Shortly thereafter, her bodily reactions and associations were indicative of primal scene derivatives, that is, of being overstimulated by an unseen instinctual object. The interpretation of *A*'s defensive effort to avoid seeing the therapist as a genital instinctual object elicited the instigating primal scene fantasy expressed in her reaction to the therapist's closed door.

Orally influenced, phallically determined representations of an object were displayed by all three patients. Infantilization was either anticipated, sought, or defended against and was accompanied by a readiness to perceive the therapist as a phallic audience or phallic humiliator. Each had a period of overdetermined closeness to, and libidinal overinvolvement with, the mother in the early phases of development. *A*'s father was away the first 2 years of her life, and she was the sole object of her mother's attention. *B* was born at a time of severe conflict between her parents and was extremely special to her mother. *C* was hovered over by her mother in the early years and left alone in dealing with the overstimulation by her father in later periods. All attempted to attain some defensive distance from the effects of this infantile attachment to the mother: *A* with an attitude of contempt for the maternal figure; *B* and *C* by directing perceptual attention to maternal deprivations.

Optimally frustrating impressions of an object are diminished, which tends to intensify a compensatory search for and struggle against infantilizing interactions. Simultaneously, these same interactions are perceived as a potential source of phallic overstimulation. When the therapist did too much or responded defensively to this pressure, he was experienced as equivalent to the distorted figures of the transference and was distrusted. When optimally frustrating responses were offered, they had the effect of amplifying dormant ego functions, enhanced integrative processes, and facilitated therapeutic progress. This was most noticeable in *A* and *B*. *A* exerted pressure on the therapist to respond, seeking reinforcement of a pathological defense. The therapist's silence strengthened her capacity to express the instinctual derivatives necessary for an interpretive intervention to be effective. *B* sought reassurance from the therapist to ease the prohibitions that dominated her internal life. The therapist's interpretation of the underlying instinctual experience was optimally frustrating, amplified her ability to form derivatives, and lessened the need for a prohibitive response. In *C*, it was displayed in a more subtle form. The therapist's silence had a defensive aspect that she unconsciously perceived. When this was acknowledged and rectified, it became possible for the transference fantasies at the foundation of her ''seductive'' behavior to emerge. All three exhibited transferences reflecting these orally influenced, phallically determined qualities. *B*, for example, was consistently concerned with the therapist's phallic characteristics. It was expressed derivatively in many teasing references to the therapist's head, which she had described as firm and solid with a bare spot on top that drew her attention. She also saw the therapist as a source of oral supplies, which was reflected in repeated requests for food.

A anticipated being humiliated by the therapist when she experienced body sensations. *C* felt totally humiliated when attention was called to her exhibitionistic behavior. *B* was convinced that the therapist was silently laughing and mocking her. These phallic and genital body ego experiences were eliciting identifications with a humiliating aggressor. The resulting reaction formations altered the experience of instinctual activity, so that phallic exhibitionism became humiliating as it moved toward voyeurism. *B*'s conviction that she would not be understood or believed was sustained by this defensive identification with a phallic humiliator and indicated that anything but an unconsciously empathic response would reenforce this compensatory, pathological position. The therapeutic task was to address the underlying body ego experiences without intensifying the need for defense. When a patient perceives the therapist as a bad object, the first consideration is to determine whether depriving, impinging, or overstimulating qualities are being introduced by the therapist's mode of functioning. However, *B* stated that this was not the case. She emphasized that it made no difference whatsoever as to what the therapist said or did. *B* was preoccupied with her painful body sensations and with being attacked by humiliating responses. She did not speak of, or experience, any direct or derivative expressions of instinctual activity. The therapist thought this was what she feared he would not be able to understand and that the interpretation of her concern that her body's language would not be understood emanated from this idea. It appeared to be an aspect of her experience that was most available to the activity of unconscious perceptions and could thereby strengthen the integrative forces in her personality. *B* reacted by expressing instinctual derivatives, revealing her masturbatory impulses, and openly masturbated when the therapist made a direct statement to that effect. She then described what this instinctual act accomplished for her. It filled her with genital sensations and diminished the force of defensive opposition. The need for a reaction formation, created by identifying with a phallic aggressor, subsided, and the underlying voyeuristic experiences of phallic overstimulation were manifested in the recall of sexual play with a cousin.

The effects of the hysteric's characterological makeup upon the process of depersonification were evidenced in the composition of instinctual derivatives. The relative diminution in the activity of this process was illustrated by the degree to which derivatives remained bound to the memory traces of infantile attachments and infantile experience. In *B*, derivative expressions of masturbatory activity were reflected in her thoughts about exploring caves, jungles, and forests. These representations of body ego experiences, although depersonified, were closely linked to the original experience. In *H*, the ''hot dog'' joke was indicative of a fantasied infantile genital attachment that had been exposed to an inefficient process of depersonification. *C* also presented many derivatives only slightly removed form the representations of infantile experience.

Castration anxiety was manifested in all three patients and served regulatory and signaling functions. Castration anxiety is a structured union of the lines of continuity of instinctual and prohibitive experiences; it consolidates during the phallic and genital phases and is uniquely adapted to serve a signaling function. The anxiety focused upon the threat of being exposed as lacking or deficient, which is consonant with the girl's concern in regard to genital body ego experiences. In the boy, castration anxiety would emerge as a threat to the integrity of the genitals. Repression proper was the clearly established primary defensive activity of the ego and functioned at the level of directing perceptual attention away from the source of a potentially traumatic stimulus. The varied superego functions remained polarized and in opposition to the interests of the ego. In all three patients, efforts to engage in work, play, or love relationships were interfered with by the conflicts they engendered. Ego interests and superego responses were at variance with each other.

A felt her leg itch and directed attention to the therapist. She attempted to focus upon the therapist's not talking as the source of her discomfort. The itching was an expression of instinctual activity intermingled with defensive opposition and accompanied by anxiety. *A* was fearful of the therapist's accusation that she was masturbating, which reflected the signaling and regulatory functions of castration anxiety. Instinctual intensity increased, an identification with a humiliating aggressor was invoked, and perceptual attention was directed away from the source of stimulation. She avoided making the connection of her itching with the mounting demand for the therapist to alleviate it. The therapist's intervention had the effect of fostering integrative functions, perceptual attention was directed to the source, and a transference-based primal scene derivative was recalled. The initial anxiety in relation to the therapist's closed door was a response to the instinctual asrousal associated with the fantasy of an unseen object.

The therapist's interpretation of *B*'s defensive posture, and the underlying masturbatory wish, led to the emergence of well-regulated genital sensations. She stated that the therapist's words gave her permission. The intensity mounted, and derivatives of overstimulation and defense were expressed in the memories of voyeuristic sexual play and the red-haired guard at the tollbooth. Phallic exhibitionism, represented as an aspect of good self-experience, shifted to having voyeuristic qualities as intensity increased and defenses were instituted. Castration anxiety functioned to elicit prohibitions, which were manifested in a feeling of badness and lack of worth. Defenses had been signaled that served to repress the genital oedipal attachments that were most threatening.

The instinctual significance of *C*'s exhibitionism was rendered defensively inaccessible to her by the effects of a fixed, phallically determined manner of perceiving all stimuli. Her attention was totally focused upon defensive responses, as instinctual experiences were enacted in her behavior. The therapist's silence was unconsciously perceived by her as defensive and, hence, was a cause for distrust. The therapist's interpretation made *C* aware of the instinctual experience she was expressing and immediately activated a reaction formation based on an identification with a humiliating aggressor. The emerging voyeuristic impulses were then replaced by an intense feeling of exposure and humiliation. The effects created by repressed representations of phallic overstimulation were then manifested in her fantasy of the therapist's arousal. Derivative associations revealed the foundation upon which her fixed character attitudes and perceptions were based.

Defense transferences in the female hysteric are based upon a negative oedipal configuration. This was not so evident in the vignettes protrayed but emerged in all three patients in the course of their therapeutic experiences. *A*, for example, displayed much conscious contempt for what she described as her mother's inept efforts to care for her, which barely concealed an underlying instinctual attachment. Similarly, whenever the therapist intervened, *A* experienced it as infantilizing. Her attitude was of contempt, again barely concealing the instinctual attachment. This is one of the areas where the sex of the therapist appears to have an influence on the emerging transference. Were the therapist a woman, the instinctual aspect might be more available. The therapist, in being a man, presented a greater threat because instinctual experience resonated with the representation of the male as an unseen genital instinctual object. In the hysteric with symptoms, the introjective arm of perception is periodically open to register new experiences, and the therapist's gender may have more of an effect. With character pathology, the actual gender of the therapist is probably less of a factor.

The conscious and preconscious systems of mental activities (in *A, B,* and *C*) displayed the increase in imagery and body sensations and in the diminution in immediate perceptions and projective processes that are characteristic of hysterical pathology. Drive development reflected the uneven distribution in libidinal representations, with a predominance of orally influenced, phalically determined experience. Aggression was differentiating in its effects. A hypersensitivity to, and readiness for, genital overstimulation was displayed by all three patients.

The differences between hysterical character pathology and hysterical symptom formation are determined by the status of the fixation points and by the effects of fixed character attitudes upon inner experience and psychic functioning. The conscious motivation for treatment is strong in individuals with hysterical symptoms because the thrust for progressive development is active. The symptom functions as an internal regulator and allows new object-related perceptions to be registered and represented. *A* and *B* displayed a strong conscious motivation for treatment. Unconsciously, the move to establish a genital instinctual attachment to an object operated as a source of intense anxiety. With hysterical character pathology, conscious motivation for treatment is weakened by the high level of anxiety associated with the threat of exposure. This was illustrated by *C* in her description of previous therapeutic contacts, and the potential for disruption of the therapy in the example given. The unconscious motive to seek reinforcement for fixed, defensively maintained perceptions and character attitudes can be a compelling force. Pressure is then exerted upon the therapist to participate in interactions that reenforce pathological defenses. This form of participation strengthens pathological defenses, colludes with destructive forces in the patient's personality, repeats developmental traumas, and creates a cause for distrust. However, to simply abstain may result in a level of anxiety that weakens the motive for treatment. C left her previous therapies when her "seductiveness" was interpreted, which was experienced by her as evidence that the therapist was either seductive or defensive in response to the instinctual qualities of an interaction.

In the cohesive disorders, perceptual functions establish well-defined boundaries for the systems of unconscious, preconscious, and conscious mental activities, which are then in a state of reactive continuity to each other. A given interaction evokes an unconscious perception of its particular qualities, in addition to the unconscious fantasies that express unique and personal meaning. C did not experience herself as being seductive. She was expressing phallic exhibitionistic impulses in exposing her sexuality to the therapist. Inner regulation was ineffective, and this phallic instinctual activity readily became overstimulating. Had the therapist talked of her exposure immediately, the experience of humiliation would likely have been overwhelming. The therapist's silence evoked imagery of distrustable figures, reflecting the activity of her unconscious perceptions. In the silence, the therapist was processing the effects of the patient's stimulation, did not have an interpretive response available, and was to some degree defensively disengaged. It was this aspect of disengagement that C unconsciously perceived. The therapist knew that any attention directed to C's phallic exhibitionism would be experienced as a humiliation, and to view it as seductiveness would reflect a lack of understanding of her character pathology. In remaining silent, the therapist was infantilizing C and, in addition, behaving like the absent mother. When the therapist indicated an awareness of her distrust and acknowledged the unconscious perception of his silence, he was again functioning as a good object. C then was able to allow a fantasy of the therapist's being sexually aroused to enter her conscious experience and its source in the memories of her father's sexual arousal. Validation was present in a dream that C had the next night. She swas alone in a beach house. Teenagers, having a party on the beach, suddenly threatened to invade her house. They tried to enter, a man got them together, sat and talked to them, and C felt safe.

C was expressing poorly regulated phallic instinctual activities that required the prohibitive force of a defensive identification with a phallic humiliating aggressor. The resulting reaction formation, in conjunction with her fixed phallically determined attitudes, influenced the perception of all stimuli. Phallic instinctual activity readily shifted from exhibitionism to overstimulating voyeuristic qualities; this was manifested in her perceiving the therapist as sexually aroused and in her memories of a sexually excited man. *C*'s absorption with phallically determined meanings was a product of her defensively organized pathologic character structure. These fixed perceptions were designed to protect against the potential traumatic impact of genital, object-related instinctual demands.

An important dynamic in hysterical pathology involves the identification with a humiliating aggressor that is instigated by the readiness with which phallic instinctual activities become overstimulating. This process has a surface similarity to masochistic experiences and must be distinguished from them. *Masochism* refers to a specific relationship in which the object is represented as instinctual with qualities of domination and control and the self as instinctually aroused by these qualities. Masochism is an instinctual relationship, with the object of libidinal attachment having either orally or anally determined qualities. When the object is orally determined, it is manifested in a narcissistically structured personality, and when anally determined, in obsessive constellations. In hysterical pathology, self-experiences and the impressions of an object are phallically determined. A libidinal object is represented either as a phallic reflective audience, an object of voyeuristic interest, or an overstimulating genital object. The experience of humiliation does not represent an instinctual attachment but is based upon an identification with the humiliating influence of a phallic impinging object. It is invoked to regulate phallic overstimulation and is an obstacle to the expression of instinctual activity.

Humiliation, which is a predominant feature in the pathology of hysteria, must be distinguished from the other disorders in which it occurs. These include the narcissistic personality disorders, borderline personalities, and schizophrenias displaying compensatory distortions in self-experience. It is a manifestation of the effects of defensive responses to instinctual self-experiences that are inadequately regulated. In hysteria, this involves phallic instinctual experiences, within a cohesive, object-related personality organization. The overall level of psychic organization and the nature of the instinctual experience are the determining factors in the significance of humiliation. It represents the self as inferior, damaged, helpless, and vulnerable to the disapproval of an admired impinging object and is indicative of a distortion in self-experience.

When the impressions of an object are elaborated into compensatory defensive responses, perceptual attention is focused upon the distortions that are thereby created. The level of psychic organization determines the manner in which they are manifested. In the more advanced object-related personality, it is reflected in the extensive overintellectualizations of the obsessive with symptoms or character pathology; in the narcissistic personality disorders, it is reflected in the use of idealizations, and in the borderline personality and schizophrenias, it is reflected in paranoia.

The Structural Foundation of Thought in Hysteria

This clinical example consists of a very brief segment of mental content, which will be examined for its structural foundation. The purpose is to illustrate the application of these developmental concepts in formulating the internal conditions that are necessary to produce a given thought. All vital information is omitted in order to highlight the significance of what can be implicitly determined from the composition of a communicated thought.

"I can't think. I'm trying to study for an exam and I keep seeing images of women."

Thinking is the end result of a complex interrelationship between the representations of body ego experiences and their object-impression counterparts, which are exposed to processes of symbolization and depersonification. The autonomous ego functions are an integral part of the developmental events that have to transpire for thinking to result and are essential in determining the manner in which it is manifested. The projective screen of transitional space, the capacity to contain mental contents, and the process of symbolization are all necessary preconditions. In addition, thinking requires the perceptual function of observing a mental impression and includes the process involved in forming a thought. However, it is not in and of itself an autonomous ego function. Thinking reflects the underlying representations of self-experience and of an object's influence upon which it takes place and is affected by the mental structures that unite and differentiate the two systems of representation.

The statement, "I can't think," immediately reveals that the conflict-free sphere of the ego is not involved and implies that thinking is a function available under certain conditions. The next segment, "I'm trying to study for an exam," begins to identify the conditions that interfere with the psychic activity of thinking. Self-experience is reflected in the pronoun "I" and refers to being engaged in trying to study. It represents the self's attempting to look at something to discover its significance. This perceptual activity is associated with a prohibition, and the imagery of women emerges to take its place. The exam represents the depersonification of an object, which requires a significant degree of differentiation and an established state of cohesiveness. There is interference with the pursuit of studying for an exam, and it is replaced by a different form of mental content. The ready emergence of imagery is indicative of an abundance of self-experiences available for the formation of derivatives and of limitations in the process of depersonification. The act of studying for an exam is prohibited, hinting at its erotization, and perceptual attention is drawn to the less threatening imagery of women. These modes of functioning appear consonant with the structural organization of the hysteric.

The shift in perceptual attention, from a prohibited attachment to a depersonified object to a less threatening attachment to women, appears to be a manifestation of the early stages of repression proper. It implies a negative oedipal constellation and tends to identify the patient as a woman. We can speculate that the thought is founded upon the representation of a prohibited instinctual attachment to a male, symbolized and depersonified into the act of studying for an exam. We can further infer that the oedipal conflict is unresolved and that the effort to displace genital instinctual interest to the male is imbued with an inordinate degree of conflict. The response is to defensively regress to a negative oedipal position, which prevents growth and learning. This speculation is descriptive of the hysterical character. The implication that studying can take place, under certain conditions, indicates that the introjective arm of perception can be open to new object-related experiences. This hints at the presence of hysterical symptoms. An individual with a hysterical character makeup and an open system of perception is vulnerable to overstimulation, and the compromises formed by a symptom provide a degree of regulation.

The thought was communicated in the context of a therapeutic relationship and has some bearing on the qualities of the interaction. When the conditions of psychotherapy are impinging, depriving, or overstimulating, the communicated thoughts will be based upon representations reflecting these qualities as derivatives of unconscious perceptions. When the conditions are unconsciously empathic, the communicated thoughts are expressive of the transference fantasy distortions arising out of developmental conflict. This thought, in being based upon representations reflecting the impact of instinctual stimuli from the interior, suggests that the therapeutic interaction possesses the qualities of a good object.

The Structural Foundation of Thought in Other Disorders

In concluding this discussion of hysteria, I would like to present a brief clinical example of a dream. Once again, all information will be omitted, to focus attention upon what can be implicitly determined from the structure of a segment of mental content. It is presented to illustrate the absence of hysterical lines of development, although the dreamer had many conversion symptoms.

"I was on my way to an airplane. I had left the terminal and was in a train that went from the terminal to the plane. I thought the plane was going to be blown up but, instead, terrorists blew up the terminal. I was relieved that I had left the terminal. The train I was in started to get out of control; I pulled the emergency brakes; the train stopped; and I woke up."

The manifest content embodies an airplane, a terminal and a vehicle transporting the dreamer from one to the other. In being a dream, the mental content is highly symbolized.

The system of self-representations is the source of all experience, and we can postulate that the terminal is a symbolic reflection of its functional activity. The terminal possesses the characteristic of being a stationary structure where things begin and end, which is consonant with the self-representational system.

The impressions of an object can be represented as a focus of interest, as a source of supply or attack, as elusive or caring but not as stationary. The system of object representations has formed from the mental impressions of independent stimuli; this makes them more distant, less under control, and more susceptible to the effects of fantasy distortions. The airplane appears to symbolically reflect the functional activity of this system of representations.

The characteristic of instinctual activity is impulsion, and the train connecting the terminal to the airplane is portrayed as in the process of that symbolic movement. The manifest content of the dream depicts an instinctual movement from the self-representational system (the terminal) to the object representational system (the airplane). This movement is reminiscent of the manner in which the grandiose self is structured.

The motivation for forming the grandiose self is the vulnerability and helplessness associated with the recognition of separateness. The purpose is to balance the experience of vulnerability by participating in the fantasied omnipotence of the object. The composition of the dream seems to express the difficulties encountered with the formation of this differentiating structure. We can speculate that pathology began to emerge at the point in development when cohesiveness was first established, with the recognition of a separate good object's influence. The manifest content of the dream seems to reflect the trauma occurring during the process of forming the grandiose self. A healthy grandiose self is the regulator of the dreaming process, and this dream is poorly regulated.

The movement from the terminal to the airplane is accompanied by the threat of an explosion, which appears to be a symbolic expression of the effects of a predominance of bad instinctual self-experience and hints at an overloading of aggression. Libido is binding in its effects when phase specific and overstimulating when excessive; aggression is differentiating when phase specific and destructive when excessive. The dream is indicative of an inordinate degree of aggression, and the form of the pathology is not along the developmental lines of hysteria.

In healthy development, the structuralization of the grandiose self is stage and phase specific. The vulnerability associated with separateness occurs during the anal period, when good instinctual self-experiences of mastery and control are in the ascendency and the impressions of a good instinctual object are elaborated into fantasies of omnipotence. This union is structured to provide a perfect match to balance the experience of vulnerability. The resulting depletion in adaptive capacities motivates the formation of the ego ideal, which is based upon selective identifications. Deficient self-potentials are elaborated into fantasies that are linked to the influences of an object that are needed to reestablish restraint and stability. The impressions of an optimally frustrating good object are exactly what is needed and are included within self-experience.

The dreamer has symbolized an explosion in the terminal but first had the idea that it would be in the airplane. It suggests the fantasy of an object filled with aggression and hints that what is needed from the influences of an object is the powerful force of counteraggression. This further delineates the absence of hysterical pathology. The train is depicted as getting out of control, creating the necessity for pulling on the emergency brakes; this is a reference to the institution of more effective defenses. We can hypothesize that the process of identification with the aggressor is not yet available to establish control and prohibition and that the superego has not consolidated its precursors into a functioning structure. The only defensive functions accessible to the dreamer to stop the instinctual activity that is getting out of control are the structured remnants of reactions to impingement and the function of self-observation effected by the eye of consciousness. This is symbolized as putting on the emergency brakes, and the perceptual activity of the eye of consiousness in a waking state is invoked. Although the clinical picture included conversion symptoms, the underlying structures reveal a narcissistic organization and an absence of object-related perceptions. The composition of the manifest dream thoughts was not consistent with a diagnosis of hysteria.

CHAPTER 5

Obsessive Character Pathology and Obsessive Symptom Formation
Preoedipal Determinants

Introduction—The Role of Aggression

An instinct is defined by the mental impressions that are available for its representation. The stimuli of instinctual demands exert their effect at the interior of the personality, are registered by the perceptual processes, and activate the representational and organizational functions of the ego. The interdependent interrelationship that evolves between perceptual functions and the resulting mental representations determines the particular nature of instinctual activity.

Body ego experiences are represented and organized into a functional system of self-representations, and their object-impression counterparts are represented and organized into a functional system of object representations. The body ego experience of perceptual contact with the intrauterine environment is represented as the background object of primary identification and serves as the original object of libidinal attachment. It represents a connection to an object that is simultaneously inside of and independent of the self, provides a background for the building of mental structure, and reflects the initial experience of phase-specific instinctual gratification. This representation expresses the essence of the binding function of libido.

Instinctual demand is on a continuum of intensity that is represented as an aspect of good self-experience when defenses are not required and as an aspect of bad self-experience with mounting intensity and the institution of defense. Overstimulating libidinal activity is associated with frustration, which is differentiating in its effects when in balanced proportions. The level of frustration reflects the degree of fusion of the libidinal and aggressive drives. Any experience of phase-specific instinctual gratification requires the restraining influence of an optimal level of frustration. In health, and to a large extent in the hysteric, the frustration represented as aggression within bad self-experience is well regulated and has a differentiating effect. The representations of bad self-experience are essential for enabling defensive functions and facilitating separation and individuation. Their object-impression counterparts are also vital for regulatory and prohibitive functions and for the development of the superego. Optimal frustration represents aggression that is well regulated and expresses the essence of differentiation.

In its extremes, aggression is no longer differentiating, but impinging, attacking, and destructive, especially of the unifying function of libidinal activity. Aggression, in excess, is destructive to cohesiveness and to the consolidation of the various aspects of self-experience into a unified entity. The background object of primary identification is represented *in utero* and serves as the background upon which all mental structure evolves. Empathic responsiveness in an interaction is evocative of and builds upon this self-representation, and a psychological symbiosis is dependent upon the firmness of its presence. The advanced developmental tasks accomplished by the neurotic require that it be solidly established, and more severe disturbances result when it is deficient or faulty. The importance of this early background structure is emphasized, because obsessive pathology involves an overloading of aggression and a relative paucity in the representation of good instinctual self-experience. These are also factors, though to a much greater degree, in more severe forms of pathology.

Object-related, cohesive forms of pathology (hysteric and obsessive), either by the strength of hereditary givens or in response to interactional processes that facilitate structure building, have experienced sufficient optimal gratification and optimal frustration to attain separation–individuation, object constancy, cohesiveness, and continuity of experience. The structural preconditions and the genital fantasies of the oedipal conflict have accomplished the shift from narcissism to object relatedness, but object-related experiences are a source of trauma rather than enhancement.

An exploration of the development of the obsessive is also an exploration of the effects of aggression represented as destructive. It is the most advanced structural organization manifesting an excess of aggression, and the mental structures that are formed reflect the inadequate fusion of aggressive and libidinal drives. In health and in the hysteric, aggression is bound, well regulated, and manifested in the functioning of defensive structures. The early development of the potential obsessive is characterized by a relative paucity of optimally gratifying interactions. The resulting excessive degree of frustration reflects the predominance of aggressive components that are inadequately neutralized. Well-regulated and neutralized aggression is the motive force behind individuation, and when poorly regulated, it is potentially traumatic and can no longer be effective in those functions. Libidinal activity is binding and provides the mechanism by which fusion with the aggressive aspect of instinctual demands can occur. A balanced proportion of good and bad qualities must be represented in order to negotiate the tasks of advancement in psychic structuralization. In health, there is an orderly, sequential, regulated process of progression. In pathology, there is an imbalance that affects the evolving mental structures and influences the perception of stimuli.

The aggressive drives serve a vital function in the process of separation–individuation and differentiation and are an integral aspect of defensive functions. They play a significant role in obsessional pathology because they are not well regulated, affect the composition of differentiating structures, and shape the configuration of the oedipal conflict. The quality of instinctual activity is best described as sadistic, reflecting the inadequate fusion of the aggressive and libidinal drives.

Early Influences in the Development of the Obsessive

The early development of the obsessive with symptoms or character pathology is characterized by a relative sparsity in phase-specific instinctual gratification during the oral period, accompanied by an overabundance of sensory stimulation in other modalities. The experience of frustration is excessive, and the amplification and use of autonomous ego functions are overemphasized. The consequence is in an imbalance in the system of self-representations, with compensatory effects in the system of object representations. Good oral instinctual self-experience is deficient, the activity of autonomous ego functions hypertrophied, instinctual overstimulation is disproportionately enlarged and dominated by an overloading of aggression, and reactions to impingement and sensory deprivations are relatively diminished. The deficiencies evolving in the self-system are compensated for by an over-elaboration in fantasy of the impressions of an object. These may take the form of idealizations or of exaggerating the object's omnipotence and sadism. This is in contrast to the individual with hysterical pathology, who has been libidinally overstimulated and sensorily deprived. The focus of attention has been so one dimensional that other aspects of sensory stimulation have been neglected. With the obsessive, the stimulation of libidinal interactions is diminished, whereas other sensory modalities are overamplified.

The effects of these early experiences are operative as separation–individuation is negotiated and instinctual expansion moves toward the period of anality. The anal phase places an indelible stamp on the developing obsessive's character structure that affects all further instinctual expansion. The configuration of representations that have been evolving lay the groundwork for this profound anal influence. In the self-system of representations, good instinctual experience is sparse, the autonomous ego functions are overdeveloped, sadism is excessive, and sensory deprivations minimal. In the object system of representations, there is a paucity of optimal gratification, and frustrating prohibitive impressions are exaggerated. The inadequate fusion of the aggressive drives has affected the impinging impressions of an object, so that they are more archaic and sadistically threatening.

The Differentiating Structures Maintaining Cohesiveness

The inordinate degree of frustration motivates the process of separation–individuation to be set in motion prematurely, and the search for a separate good object's influence is initiated late in the oral period. Although the representations of a good object are relatively deficient, the capacity to achieve this recognition is enhanced by the overdevelopment of the autonomous ego functions. The good object's bad qualities are perceived very early in the anal phase, which expands the boundaries of the self by forming two arms of perception and a focused area of internally directed perceptual activity and establishes a connection between the self- and object systems of representation. The recognition of the good object's bad anal qualities, through the line of continuity of prohibitive experience, forms a fixation point on the projective arm of perception. Object constancy is anchored, and the experience of vulnerability associated with separateness is extreme to the point of being traumatic. This premature discovery of separateness occurs at a time when the impinging impressions of a bad object are archaically anal and sadistic, which intensifies the narcissistic injury of feeling helpless. The more there is advancement into the anal phase, the more these sadistic qualities are modulated. The early body ego experiences of anality are expulsive in nature, whereas later experiences gradually include the capacity for containment and retention. The developing obsessive recognizes the representation of an early, expulsive, archaic and sadistic object. Confronted with managing this overloading of aggression, with representations of deprivation and reactions to impingement being diminished and not as available to serve a defensive function, the tendency is to utilize the autonomous ego functions defensively, further exaggerating their overdevelopment. The helplessness and vulnerability, in being extreme, creates a sense of urgency and desperation that affects the manner in which differentiating structures are formed.

The grandiose self is structured, much in the manner occurring in healthy development, and balances the extreme vulnerability associated with separateness to some extent. This unifying and differentiating structure forms early in the anal phase, when good instinctual experiences are of mastery and control and the impressions of a good instinctual object are elaborated into fantasies of omnipotence. The structuralization of this linkage occupies good instinctual self-experience with the fantasied omnipotence of an object, depleting its availability for adaptive functions and furthering the already existence imbalance in the self-system. The overloading of aggression is poorly regulated and exerts a constant demand for perceptual attention. The self-representational system does not have sufficient stability to delay, maintain regulation and control, and the eruption of poorly contained aggression is threatened. It is at this juncture that the developing obsessive encounters serious difficulties. The formation of the grandiose self, in depleting the representations of good instinctual self-experience, has initiated a potential state of trauma. The emergence of anal sadistic aggression threatens the ability to maintain mastery and control and places the stability of the grandiose self in jeopardy. The need is for an immediate defensive response, and the existing conditions lead to the emergence of pathological structures. The previous events are the precursors of, and operate as a foundation for, pathological developments. Stage and phase specificity is such an important aspect that even a small degree of a lack in synchrony can have a profound effect.

The depletion in good instinctual self-experience motivates the formation of another unifying and differentiating structure to provide regulation, balance, and stability. This structure, the ego ideal, is based upon a process of selective identification. Deficient self-potentials are elaborated into fantasies and linked to needed and admired influences of an object, which are then included within self-experience. In health, there is sufficient stability for this process to be discriminating and selective, and the ego ideal is gradually structured with movement into the phallic phase. In the developing obsessive, the conditions leading to a premature process of separation–individuation and premature structuralization of the grandiose self have become intensified. The overabundance of aggression that had been held in a precarious balance now is on the verge of flooding the self-system of representations. The structure of the ego ideal must form, not only prematurely, but rapidly as an emergency measure. The impressions of an object are sought that can provide the wherewithal to manage the aggression that is getting out of control. Intense prohibitive, controlling, and restraining influences are required for the strong counteraggressive force necessary to accomplish that task. The line of continuity of prohibitive experience, represented as optimal frustration in the good object and shading into the impingements of a bad object, is available and responsive to this need for a powerful prohibitive, counteraggressive force. The ego ideal utilizes the anally sadistic, impinging impressions of an object as an essential facet of its composition. In healthy development, this process of identification with an aggressor only occurs transiently, at times of stress or overstimulation.

In health, the experience of helplessness and vulnerability associated with separateness and the narcissistic injury it entails can be absorbed. The grandiose self provides balance, and the ego ideal strengthens adaptive capacities and integrative functions. Identifications with an aggressor and the reaction formations they create occur only transiently and are not extreme. A fixation point is formed on the introjective arm of perception during the phallic period, which provides enough stability for the structure of castration anxiety to organize and consolidate. The conditions are then present for the genital fantasies of the oedipal conflict to flourish. It is an orderly and sequential set of events that moves through the various periods of psychosexual development in a stage- and phase-specific manner, as the component instincts expand and consolidate into a genital drive.

The experience of helplessness and vulnerability associated with separateness is greater in the obsessive, and the capacity to absorb narcissistic injuries is limited. The grandiose self provides some measure of balance but, in the process, disturbs the already tenuous regulation of instinctual activity. The ego ideal is structured rapidly during the anal period and includes the sadistic impinging qualities of a bad object within self-experience. Although the frustrating influences of an object are amply available, the situation is urgent and requires more forceful restraint. Optimally frustrating qualities are needed, admired, and do offer some limited restraint. However, they depend upon evoking resources within the self-system, and these functions have been overwhelmed by the intensity of aggression. The autonomous ego functions are already overdeveloped and do not provide effective regulation. This is a major dilemma for the developing obsessive. The structure of the ego ideal is formed prematurely during the anal period, dominated by the need for the effective control of anal sadistic impulses, and include the qualities of an overcontrolling, sadistic object.

The line of continuity of instinctual experience is accentuated by the constant demand for perceptual attention exerted by the aggressive drives. In conjunction with the formation of the ego ideal, perceptual attention is directed into the self-system, and there is an immediate recognition of the good self's bad qualities. This establishes a fixation point on the introjective arm of perception prematurely, during the period of anality. Some semblance of stability is created, the control that was previously so ineffective has now appeared possible to attain, and every effort is expended to reenforce this defensive position. This is seen clinically when a therapist is admired after being provoked into responding sadistically; this serves to reenforce the obsessive's character defenses.

The Fixation Points in the Obsessive

The recognition of a separate good object's influence establishes a differentiated connection to the object system of representations. The recognition of the good object's bad qualities ensures that differentiation will be sustained and anchors object constancy. The memory trace of that infantile attachment to an object forms a fixation point, which has an effect upon the way all subsequent attachments are experienced. This fixation point, on the projective arm of perception, must expand by including progressively advanced representations of an object's good and bad qualities. Ultimately, it is depersonified so as to be free of a narcissistic influence. The obsessive forms this fixation point prematurely, with the transition into the anal period, when there has been no time or opportunity to modulate the sadistic impressions of an object. The early anal phase is characterized by expulsive qualities, reflecting the inadequate fusion of the aggressive and libidinal drives, and is intensified by the excessive aggression of the oral period. The precocious negotiation of separation–individuation cannot be initiated until the representations of good self-experience are sufficiently consolidated and structuralized at the interior to buffer the impact of biophysiological demands. The early recognition of a separate good object's influence, made possible by the overdevelopment of the autonomous ego functions, occurs slightly out of stage and phase specificity. In health, the fixation point forms later in the anal period, when the retentive qualities reflecting an increased capacity to bind, regulate, and control anal sadistic experiences have emerged.

Although the grandiose self is formed prematurely, and the experience of vulnerability associated with separateness heightened, the significance of these events is primarily manifested in the evolution of pathology with the formation of the ego ideal. The composition of this structure is determined by an excessive need for the prohibitive influences of an object and is based upon the identification with an anal-sadistic aggressor. This advancing step in differentiation is accompanied by an abrupt and premature recognition of the good self's bad instinctual qualities. A fixation point is established on the introjective arm of perception, based upon the memory traces of anal-sadistic instinctual experience, which is rigid and inflexible. In health, the line of continuity of instinctual experience is perceived as a gradual blending of instinctual activities from those that do not require defense into the emergence of defense with mounting intensity. In the obsessive, it is an abruptly demarcated transition with no gradation. The presence of tenacious, anally determined fixation points on both the projective and introjective arms of perception exerts a strong distorting effect upon succeeding advancements in instinctual representation. The anality of the potential obsessive is thereby secured.

The fixation point on the introjective arm of perception exerts an anally derived influence upon all stimuli and is at the foundation of obsessive character pathology. When the resulting fixed character attitudes are ineffective in sustaining repression, this fixation point may be regressively relinquished. The force of the aggressive drives, in overcoming defensive opposition, has created a breakdown in its function. This generally occurs under conditions of stress or trauma, and obsessive symptoms develop in an effort to regulate what has become an open system of perception by the formation of compromises. The symptoms reflect a frantic attempt to manage the influx of instinctual overstimulation in the internal world and the stimuli of new experiences in the external world. The degree of stress threatens the state of cohesiveness and mobilizes the anxiety of fragmentation. In the hysteric, an open system of perception is indicative of a developmental advance with some degree of oedipal conflict resolution. The character pathology of hysteria is invoked as a defensive and regressive move. In the obsessive, an open system of perception and the formation of symptoms are the result of an ineffectiveness in the defensive function of character pathology.

The process of identification with a sadistic aggressor has mobilized the prohibitive influences of a bad impinging object so that they are operative within the realm of self-experience. The demand for perceptual attention exerted by sadistic instinctual activities elicits the response created by that identification. The experience is then perceived as disgust, shame, or guilt, depending upon the urgency with which an identification has been made and the degree to which the sadistic influences of an object have been modulated. This is at the foundation of the reaction formations that are a predominant feature of the obsessive's development.

The Nature of Reaction Formations

Reaction formations are the beginning stage of consolidating the precursors of the superego into an independently functioning regulatory and guiding agency. The process of identification with an aggressor eventuates in the reaction formations that instigate changes in the experience of instinctual activity. This defensively organized response, to instinctual overstimulation, lays the groundwork for the effectiveness of repression proper.

The line of continuity of instinctual experience expands in accordance with the evolution of the component instincts. In conjunction with the formation of the ego ideal, a structured pathway is available for including within self-experience those influences of an object that provide more effective regulation of instinctual demands. In health, the ego ideal is primarily based upon identifications with the qualities of a good object. At moments of stress, or increased instinctual stimulation, the greater prohibitive force offered by the impressions of a bad object is available for transient identifications. These identifications with an aggressor establish a clear demarcation between instinctual experiences that do not require defense and those that are overstimulating. Instinctual demands necessitating defense mobilize the prohibitive responses attained by identification with an aggressor, and the resulting reaction is perceived. A change is thereby created in the manner in which overstimulating instinctual demands are experienced.

In the obsessive, identifications with an anally determined aggressor are more permanent, as a consequence of the constant pressure from the overactivity of sadistic impulses. The reaction formations they create alter the perception of these bad instinctual self-experiences, and the response of disgust, shame, or guilt are noted in their stead. These reaction formations, in carrying the prohibitive influences of an object into the realm of self-experience, are the earliest stages of superego organization. They occur in tandem with the emergence of repression proper as the primary defensive activity of the ego. Initially, superego functions are polarized, with the idealizing functions organizing within the system of object representations and the prohibitive functions organizing within the system of self-representations. Repression proper operates to direct perceptual attention away from the source of threatening stimuli.

In health, the final stage of superego consolidation is achieved through selective identifications, in conjunction with the resolution of the oedipal conflict. The result is in an integration of superego functions operating in harmony with the interests of the ego, and repression proper directing perceptual attention to the source of a given stimulus. In hysteria, reaction formations are specifically in response to phallic overstimulation. Superego organization begins with the process of identification with a phallic humiliating aggressor, and the degree of consolidation is dependent upon the degree to which the oedipal conflict is resolved. When there is sufficient progression to attain regulation through the formation of symptoms, there is some degree of resolution of the oedipal conflict, some degree of integration of the fixation point on the introjective arm of perception, and some degree of superego consolidation. With hysterical character pathology, there is a lack of resolution of the oedipal conflict, the fixation point on the introjective arm of perception remains unintegrated, the superego remains at an immature level of organization, and repression proper directs perceptual attention away from a source of stimulation.

The obsessive emphasizes reaction formations created prematurely by identification with an archaic, sadistic aggressor and remains at an immature stage of superego organization. Anally derived reaction formations are a more permanent part of the obsessive's character structure, having an affect upon all continuing advancements in development. Perceptual attention is focused upon good anal instinctual experiences of mastery and control, as poorly fused libidinal and aggressive drives are constantly defended against. The obsessive finds it mandatory to develop fixed character attitudes that both amplify these good instinctual qualities and reinforce reaction formations. The fixed attitudes, designed to adapt to the demands of the internal and external worlds, exert anal-sadistic control over all objects and exaggerate the sense of mastery and autonomy. Although they are often seen by others as hostile and sadistic, they are not perceived this way by the obsessive. The conscious experience of sadistic impulses threatening to emerge is of disgust, shame, or guilt, and aggression is only perceived in the external world.

The obsessive utilizes repression but not effectively. Each stimulus is a potential purveyor of the instinctual activity that must be warded off, and reaction formations give expression to the sadism that is being reacted against. A reaction formation goes beyond the experiences of believing in the validity of a perception. A belief is modifiable by interpretation through the perceptual activities of the eye of consciousness and the integrative functions of the conscious system. Reaction formations are based on a structural alteration in the experience of a stimulus and are relatively unmodified solely by interpretive interventions.

The Effects of the Obsessive's Development upon Thinking, Perception, and Adaptation

The constant potential for loss of control, especially of aggressive impulses, heightens the sensitivity to these qualities in others and narrows the range and scope of relationships. The sensitivity is a combination of a reactive familiarity with aggressive stimuli and an overdevelopment of projective processes. Over intellectualization and a hypercathexis of conscious mental contents characterize the thinking style of the obsessive, which is a direct consequence of the defensive effort to master instinctual demands through the use of autonomous ego functions. The mechanism of isolation, associated with the repression of instinctual activity, is necessary for the ego function of concentration. In the obsessive, it is accentuated and highly overdeveloped. Processes of depersonification gain little independence from the influence of infantile attachments to an object, and fixed, anally determined perceptions stand in opposition to the organization of a conflict-free system of mental functioning. The obsessive's character is constructed to ensure control and to maintain an unawareness of anal-sadistic impulses. The fixation point on the introjective arm of perception is defensively maintained, giving an anally determined coloration to all further instinctual expansion. The structural preconditions necessary for an oedipal conflict to evolve are formed during the pregenital phases of development and affect the oedipal conflict itself to a degree that makes object-related perceptions a source of trauma. The impact of anal-sadistic aggression upon these developing structures in such that the stabilizing presence of a fixation point on the introjective arm of perception cannot be relinquished. Object-related perceptions, in being traumatic rather than enhancing, must be defended against. The unseen objects in the external world and their representation in the internal world are a potential source of danger.

CHAPTER 6

Obsessive Character Pathology and Obsessive Symptom Formation
Oedipal Determinants

Introduction—The Anal Influence in Obsessive Disorders

The stimuli of impingements occur at the point of perceptual contact with the external world and from the impact of instinctual demands at the interior. The impingements of the external world are registered and shaped by their evocative connection to the instinctual impingements at the interior. The impinging impressions of an object are thereby represented in accordance with the phase of psychosexual development that is in the ascendency. The reactions to these impingements, represented as an aspect of bad self-experience, are nondiscriminatory.

In the developing obsessive, there has been a relative paucity in external impingements and a concurrent intensification of instinctual impingements. The excessive degree of frustration has served to amplify an overdevelopment of autonomous ego functions and has motivated a premature process of separation–individuation. The recognition of separateness occurs early in the anal period and is anchored by the awareness of a good object's bad anal qualities. The fixation point that is then established on the projective arm of perception is based upon the anal-sadistic influences of an impinging object.

Reactions to impingement, which aid in defending against overstimulation, are somewhat limited and affect the capacity for instinctual representation. The balance between anal instinctual self-experiences of mastery and control that do not require defense and the anal-sadistic experiences necessitating a defensive response is narrow and poorly controlled. The grandiose self is structured to balance the vulnerability associated with separateness, involves participation in a fantasy of the object's omnipotence, and disturbs the already tenuous balance of instinctual activity. The ego ideal is structured prematurely during the anal period, under emergency conditions, in an effort to restore regulation. It is based primarily on identifications with the anal-sadistic influences of an object and leads to an early recognition of the good self's bad anal instinctual qualities. The resulting fixation point formed on the introjective arm of perception establishes a fixed anal cast to the perception of all stimuli. The component instincts continue to expand, and all further representation of phallic and genital body ego experiences are affected by this fixed anal perspective. Castration anxiety consolidates the lines of continuity of instinctual and prohibitive experiences into an anally influenced genital structure.

The structuralization of cohesiveness has linked the varied systems of consciousness each to the other, so that the mental activity in one system reverberates throughout the entire personality. Instinctual demand and unconscious mental activity mobilize a myriad of derivatives registered by the focused areas of perceptual functioning in the preconscious and conscious systems. Conversely, immediate perceptions registered in the conscious system resonate with the mental contents of the preconscious and unconscious systems. Although the obsessive characteristically focuses attention upon conscious mental activity, there is an evocative connection to the representations of anally determined experiences that continue to exert their influence. The developing obsessive registers phallic and genital sensations, but they are affected by an underlying anal fixation.

The degree of pathology in the obsessive disorders is in direct proportion to the amount of modulation of anal sadism that has been developmentally attained. The range is from the most expulsive to the most controlling. The more there is movement into the anal period before the unifying and differentiating structures of the grandiose self and ego ideal are formed, the more that sadistic control is represented. The foundations of pathology are initiated in these pregenital phases of development and are manifested with the elaboration of an oedipal conflict. The obsessive disorders are object related; this signifies that the capacity for registering and representing the stimuli of independent objects and the stimuli of the unseen dimension of biophysiological demand have evolved. A structured pathway for the integration of instinctual demand and a new object-related boundary for the unconscious system have formed at the interior. The initial step of including the unseen dimension of instinctual demands within the system of self-representations has been negotiated. The further step of instinctual integration leading to sublimation and secondary autonomy remains largely unavailable. The period of pubescence and adolescence has not resulted in a replacement of the representations of primary infantile attachments to an object, the oedipal conflict is unresolved, and the superego is in its earliest stages of organization. The fixation point on the projective arm of perception is overdeveloped as a compensatory measure, under the dominance of an infantile anally determined attachment to an object. The fixation point on the introjective arm of perception is tenaciously maintained under the dominance of infantile anal instinctual experience. The process of depersonification is not free of these infantile influences, and the conflict-free sphere has not evolved into a system of functions. All mental activity is occupied with the expression of, and defense against, the effects of an anally determined genital oedipal conflict.

The Preconditions for the Oedipal Conflict and the Structure of Castration Anxiety

The premature establishment of anally determined fixation points, on both the projective and introjective arms of perception, has a profound effect upon the structures that form as preconditions for the oedipal conflict. In health, the fixation point on the projective arm is formed well into the anal period; the grandiose self and ego ideal are structured in a stage- and phase-specific manner; and a fixation point is formed on the introjective arm of perception late in the phallic phase. The orderly sequence of structuralization allows the representation of progressive pregenital attachments to an object to anchor object constancy and expand the fixation point on the projective arm of perception. The fixation point on the introjective arm is maintained long enough to offer the stability necessary for castration anxiety to be structured and for the genital fantasies of the oedipal conflict to exert their organizing effect. The period of fixed perceptions is transient and readily relinquished, as the capacity for object-related perceptions is created and the oedipal conflict resolved. The shift from narcissism to object relatedness is negotiated; new object-related structures are formed; and there is an increased ability to represent greater intensities of instinctual demand. Any further increase in instinctual activity serves as an impetus for further self-expansion.

In the obsessive, the need for stability and regulation is so urgent that the fixation points are formed prematurely and are defensively maintained. There is sufficient structuralization for further instinctual expansion to occur and for the progressive thrust of development to continue. However, the premature anal fixation leaves an imprint on the body ego experiences and object impressions that are subsequently represented. Phallic and genital instinctual experiences are perceived as having anally sadistic qualities, and the phallic and genital impressions of an object are registered as having anal attributes. These anal-genital qualities are incorporated in the structure of castration anxiety, shape the configuration of oedipal fantasies, and contribute to the traumatic impact of object-related perceptions.

Castration anxiety is structured during the period of genital consolidation by uniting the lines of continuity of prohibitive and instinctual experiences. It embodies the representation of an instinctual self opposed by the restraining or threatening force of a prohibitive object and is a necessary precondition for the elaboration of an oedipal conflict. This structure is organized to provide the regulatory function required in negotiating the transition from narcissisim to object relatedness. A signaling function is possible because both good and bad qualities of the self and object are included in its composition. In the developing obsessive, castration anxiety is an archaic, harshly punitive, anally sadistic, castrating structure because the increase in instinctual intensity associated with the oedipal conflict mobilizes this prohibitive response.

The Oedipal Conflict in the Obsessive

The development of object-related perceptions is an integral part of, and dependent upon, the formation of an oedipal conflict. The new structures that are created establish a foundation for registering and representing the unseen dimension on the continuum of biophysiological demand in the internal world and for recognizing the independent qualities of an object in the external world. The manner in which the oedipal conflict forms and its fate are crucial in determining the effects and significance of these object-related experiences.

The early development of the potential obsessive has eventuated in a fixed anal perspective, which has obviated against the internalization of new experiences. The anal coloration that is exerted upon all stimuli (both inner and outer) affects the expansion of instinctual activity into phallic components and the eventual consolidation into a genital drive. There is an increasing awareness of phallic and genital body ego sensations, but they are represented with the distorting effects of a fixated, anally influenced perceptual attitude. The mental structures that maintain cohesiveness and provide stability and regulation all reflect this effect of anality.

The anal-genital consolidation of the component instincts and the elaboration of oedipal fantasies take place with the threatening prohibitive force of castration anxiety as a constant presence. The increased instinctual activity associated with the oedipal conflict is accompanied by an effort to master its effects through the use of overdeveloped processes of intellectualization. The object-related experiences of the obsessive are not enhancing as they are in healthy development, or alternately enhancing and overstimulating as they are in the hysteric, but are a source of sadistic attack or control that can reach traumatic proportions. The ancillary defensive unions, composed of the representations of impingements and deprivations, are relatively underdeveloped and do not operate effectively.

Primal scene fantasies, reflecting the structured pathway of instinctual integration, are a source of anal-genital instinctual attacks. Incestuous fantasies, reflecting the new boundary for the unconscious system, express the instinctual demand for sadistic control of, and engagement with, a genitally determined object. The boundary of the unconscious system is a major defensive response and is highly accentuated. The obsessive is filled with sadistic fantasies of controlling a genital instinctual object to defend against fantasies of anal penetration by an uncontrolled (and controlling) genital instinctual object. Superego functions are dominated by the reaction formations organized during the pregenital phases of development and the ability to direct perceptual attention toward less threatening defensive constellations functions with limited effectiveness. The fixation points are defensively maintained by a tenacious attachment to the representations of infantile experience on which they are based. The fixation point on the introjective arm of perception is only relinquished with a regressive breakdown in function.

The Oedipal Conflict in the Male

The portal of entry of instinctual demand is represented as an overstimulating instinctual object. During the period of oedipal organization, it is elaborated into primal scene fantasies that are structurally linked to the representations of bad instinctual self-experience. The first step in a pathway of instinctual integration is structured, which, when well regulated, ensures a continuous flow of instinctual activity toward attaining secondary autonomy. In the developing male obsessive, this instinctual attachment to the impression of a maternal object is evocative of poorly regulated, sadistic (expulsive or controlling) genital impulses. The immediate, excessively prohibitive response is of a sadistic, castrative threat, creating an urgent need to displace instinctual interest to the male. A feminine identification becomes mandatory and the lifelong yearning for close contact with a female makes this defensive maneuver attractive. The process of identification, in not being instinctually based, permits feminine attributes to be readily included within self-experience. In this way, the frustration and sadism that are mobilized in a genital instinctual attachment are defended against. The persistent focus on anal erotogenic zones fuses anal sensations with genital stimulation, and the absence of a phallically determined overevaluation of the genital allows the symbolic relinquishment of the penis that is essential to sustain a feminine identification. This feminine identification can then serve as the basis for representing the genital as the symbolic organ of attachment to an object, received through anal penetration. The male obsessive can displace his instinctual object relatively easily as a result of the paucity in optimally gratifying experiences, the overloading of aggression, and the continuing anal influence on phallic and genital sensations.

The influences of an object can be included within self-experience at two separate locales, involving two entirely different processes. One is at the interior of the personality, when the instinctual impression of an overstimulating object is linked through its primal scene fantasy to self-experiences of genital overstimulation. This is the extension of the line of continuity of instinctual experience, structured into a pathway of integration by the oedipal conflict. In the obsessive, it is inordinately conflicted, defensively distorted into a negative oedipal constellation, and registered as anally penetrating. The second locale is at the periphery, when deficient self-potentials are elaborated in fantasy, linked to the qualities of an object that are needed and admired, and included within self-experience. In the obsessive, this process of selective identification is dominated by the need for prohibitive influences during the pregenital phases of development and by feminine identifications with an anal genital consolidation.

A negative oedipal conflict is characteristic for the male obsessive. The threat of castration is so enormous, feminine identifications and passivity so enticing, and genital instinctual activity so affected by anality that a defensive displacement of sexual interest to the male is readily adopted. In this negative oedipal position, genital instinctual demands can be included within self-experience, although with great difficulty and through the fantasy of anal penetration. The fantasy of anal penetration reflects the intensity of instinctual demand's penetrating defensive responses, indicates the absence of a regulated, integrative process, and is a more traumatic, defensively distorted, pathological version of a primal scene fantasy. In health, this structure enables a continuous flow of instinctual demand to be included within self-experience, where there is ready access to integrative functions and secondary autonomy. In hysteria, primal scene fantasies are overstimulating, partially integrated with the aid of symptomatic compromises, and blocked from gaining access to secondary autonomy when character pathology is manifested. In the obsessive, primal scene fantasies are structured to enable the representation of the unseen dimension on the continuum of instinctual demand, but these object-related perceptions are fraught with anxiety. In the male, this aspect of instinctual demand can only be included within self-experience when a defensive feminine identification has been affected.

The representations of bad genital instinctual self-experience are elaborated into incestuous fantasies, which are structurally linked to the impressions of an overstimulating instinctual object to form a new boundary for the unconscious system. In the male obsessive, these incestuous fantasies, expressing anal sadistic genital control over a forbidden object, are heavily predominant and are often accompanied by masturbation to activate their defensive function. Ancillary defensive unions organized in response to the oedipal conflict are relatively ineffective; this accentuates the need to reinforce the fixed character attitudes and reaction formations already existent. The superego remains in its early stages of organization, and perceptual attention is occupied with the compensatory defensive activity in the object representational system, with excessive intellectualizations, and with the overemphasis upon autonomous ego functions.

The Oedipal Conflict in the Female

In the female, the proximity of anal and genital sensations exaggerates the anal influence upon the expansion of the component instincts and their consolidation into a genital drive. The inadequate fusion of aggressive and libidinal drives, in conjunction with an ineffective regulation of instinctual activity, exerts a constant impulsion to alleviate excessive frustration through masturbatory acts. Reaction formations, based upon identifications with the impinging impressions of an anally sadistic object, establish intense prohibitions. There is a constant state of vigilance against the expression of these anal-genital experiences of overstimulation. The structure of castration anxiety is disproportionately prohibitive and is manifested in an anally sadistic condemnation of the female genital as defective. The oedipal fantasies are then elaborated under these difficult conditions.

In the healthy development of the female, a negative oedipal configuration is a developmental step toward displacement of genital interest to the male. The displacement is motivated by a genital disappointment in the primary nurturing maternal figure. A genital instinctual attachment to the mother cannot provide the gratifications that her body experiences demand, and genital interest is displaced to the father. The obsessive carries the effects of anality into the genital oedipal period, and the developmental step of a negative oedipal attachment is excessively traumatic. Perceiving the maternal object as the source of instinctual gratification, with its ensuing disappointment, is too evocative of the poorly controlled sadistic aggression that is already present. The representations of a male object, forming in the shadow of the primary object, are readily available for the rapid displacement of an anally influenced genital attachment. The penis is symbolically endowed with anal qualities and is perceived as an organ to be controlled and contained from within, reflecting the genital meaning that is given to anal sensations.

The new structures organized by the oedipal conflict, to establish object-related perceptions, are affected by this defensive avoidance of a negative oedipal constellation. Primal scene fantasies, reflecting the structured pathway of instinctual integration, are of anal subjugation to an overpowering, penetrating genital instinctual object. Incestuous fantasies, reflecting the new boundary for the unconscious system, involve anal control over a genital masculine object. Masculine identifications are sought as a source of strength for exerting anal control and reenforcing this defensive structure. The unseen dimension of instinctual demand is included within self-experience, but the maintenance of an anally fixated character structure prevents any further integration. The superego remains in an early stage of consolidation and directs perceptual attention to the exaggerated use of ideational functions. This is a manifestation of the effort to master instinctually based derivatives of an unresolved oedipal conflict through intellectual processes.

The Significance of Obsessive Character Pathology

The early development of the obsessive has been characterized by psychological distance rather than involvement. A balanced proportion of external impingements facilitates the representation of instinctual demands that are impinging at the interior. The excessive degree of frustration, in combination with a diminution in external impingements, is an important factor in the defensive organization that eventuates. The developing infant has had to depend too much on its own resources for managing the effects of this relatively high level of frustration. The obsessive is somewhat limited in being able to fully represent the impinging aspects of instinctual demand, and the unseen dimension is not as capable of representation, as is the case in health or in the hysteric. The hysteric has been both impinged upon and gratified a great deal and, as a result, has more capacity for mental representation. When biophysiological demands make an impact on perceptual processes in the absence of a capacity for representation, it has an unstabilizing effect. The formation of fixation points influences the manner in which stimuli are registered and provides stability at the expense of narrowing the range of perceptual experience. The obsessive has been faced with such a high degree of instability that, once the anally derived fixation points are established, they are tenaciously maintained, and there is a great reluctance to relinquish the stability they offer. In a therapeutic situation, this is one reason why silence is helpful to the hysteric and often is a deterrent to the obsessive. In addition, although impinging qualities in a therapeutic interaction are unconsciously unempathic and undesirable, the obsessive frequently indicates that they are more workable than an unempathic silence.

Character pathology is designed to defensively maintain stability by registering all stimuli on the basis of the memory traces of anally derived infantile attachments to an object and of anally sadistic instinctual experiences. Fixed attitudes are developed to reenforce the reaction formations necessary to manage the threatening anal-sadistic drives and to focus attention upon the good instinctual experiences of mastery and control and upon autonomous functioning. One characteristic of these attitudes is in the contained hostility, apparent to all but the obsessive. Their subtle, sadistic, controlling effect upon external objects often elicits an aggressive response. The obsessive reacts with bewilderment when confronted with this counteraggression, being totally unaware of how it was initiated.

The Significance of Obsessive Symptoms

When the anally determined fixation points and the reaction formations supporting their defensive function are not successful in regulating instinctual demand, the fixation point on the introjective arm of perception is regressively relinquished. This represents an attempt to attain a previously held perceptual position. The defensive function of this fixation point is no longer available, an open system of perception is regressively recreated, and instinctual activity gains expression and some degree of regulation through forming the compromises embodied in obsessive symptoms. The regression to a perceptual position established prior to the formation of a fixation point on the introjective arm of perception requires an undoing of, and disengagement from, the identifications with an anal-sadistic aggressor incorporated in the structure of the ego ideal. It is the structuralization of the ego ideal that made the recognition of the good self's bad instinctual qualities possible, and this regressive disengagement results in a loss of that perceptual capacity. Perceptual attention is no longer directed away from this source of overstimulation, but the undoing of a structure has created a lack of recognition. This regressive loss of function is motivated by the threat of being overwhelmed by the effects of uncontrolled sadistic instinctual activity. The demand for perceptual attention has been of an intensity that could no longer be controlled by maintaining the fixation point, and perceptual attention is focused almost exclusively upon the compensatory overactivity in the object system of representations.

Although there is a regressive return to a previous perceptual position, the individual is confronted with a changed set of conditions. The representations of an object now include the anal-genital instinctual and harshly punitive castrative qualities associated with the oedipal conflict. Maturbatory impulses become more insistent, as the need to activate incestuous fantasies is more acute, and they must be warded off. The mental structures at the foundation of cohesiveness and the lines of cleavage consolidating the varied facets of self-experience into defined entities are under stress from the destructive effects of poorly regulated aggression. A hierarchy of obsessive symptomatology, from ideational symptoms to compulsive rituals, emerges as a defensive solution and diminishes the threat of fragmentation. The symptom is a compromise in which anally influenced, genitally determined instinctual demands are given expression disguised by an accompanying defensive reaction; it includes the superego's prohibitive response of disgust, shame, or guilt and involves an adaptive component in exerting sadistic control over objects in the external world.

The hierarchy of symptoms that are manifested depends upon the degree to which psychic structuralization has been affected by archaic, anal sadistic qualities. The more modulation that is attained, the more the symptoms involve ideational components, and the more effective they are in providing regulation. The more that anal sadism is archaic, the necessity for symptomatic compromises to involve behavioral rituals increases. At the extreme, the symptoms encompass body ego experiences. This hierarchy of symptoms, from an emphasis upon the overactivity of the object representational system to including the realm of self-experience, from ideational activity to action, gives some indication of the degree of control over the aggressive drives. To the extent that aggression is out of control, the threat of fragmentation and the potential for self-injury and self-destruction increase. Ideational symptoms are instinctual derivatives that uncontrollably erupt into consciousness, disguised by a prohibitive defensive response, and elicit disgust, shame, or guilt. They are evocative of compulsive, repetitive efforts to undo the effects of their expression. This circular process reflects the attempt to regulate instinctual activity in an open system of perception. When it cannot be managed by ideational activity, which is more distant from immediate experience, compromises are expressed in behavioral rituals and finally bodily responses such as tics and hand-washing compulsions.

The Significance of the Defensive Organization of the Obsessive

In healthy development, the line of continuity of instinctual experience is initially perceived as a gradation, which gives flexibility to the fixation point that is formed on the introjective arm of perception. However, it must be firmly demarcated for repression proper to function effectively. It is important for a change to take place in the perception of this gradation that clearly defines the transition and maintains the necessary flexibility. The stabilizing effect of this fixation point sets in motion a sequence of developmental events in preparation for the shift from narcissism to object relatedness. This shift is organized around the oedipal conflict, is associated with a marked increase in instinctual activity, and requires a regulatory influence. Castration anxiety consolidates as a signaling and regulating structure, and the beginning stages of organizing the superego's precursors into a unified structural agency are initiated.

The evolving superego regulates, monitors, directs, and is an integral part of repression proper. The interrelationship is facilitated by more clearly defining the point at which instinctual demand requires the institution of defense. The ego ideal has structured a pathway that enables the restraining and prohibitive influences of an object to be included within self-experience. This process of selective identification creates the change by which the gradient of instinctual experience is replaced with a perception of a restraining, prohibitive response. The resulting reaction formation serves as the foundation upon which repression proper rests and is the earliest stage of superego consolidation. Healthy reaction formations are well modulated, and the restraining force of the optimally frustrating impressions of a good object are generally sufficient. Identifications with the impinging impressions of a bad object are only invoked at transient moments of stress and overstimulation. With the resolution of the oedipal conflict, the superego assumes the functions of regulation and guidance with increasing independence from external objects and from the influence of narcissistic structures. The stabilizing function of the fixation point on the introjective arm of perception is then no longer necessary, and it is relinquished as the integration of instinctual demand is more fully achieved. This process leading to secondary autonomy enlarges the realm of the conflict-free sphere of the ego, and new object-related experiences are registered in an open system of perception.

In the obsessive disorders, an anally determined fixation point on the introjective arm of perception must be defensively maintained. Reaction formations are not modulated and are based primarily on identifications with an impinging, anally sadistic aggressor. The superego remains at its earliest stages of organization. Repression proper has emerged as the major defensive activity of the ego but is ineffective and requires the reinforcement of anally derived fixation points, unmodulated reaction formations, and ideational overactivity. The oedipal conflict is unresolved, and object-related experiences are a source of trauma. When repression proper is unsuccessful, the protective response is a regressive relinquishing of the fixation point on the introjective arm of perception. Instinctual demand is then granted expression through the compromises of symptom formation, and some degree of regulation results. The obsessive disorders, though object related, are at the threshold of narcissistic forms of pathology.

A structured pathway of instinctual integration requires the negotiation of two distinct developmental tasks. The first is to structuralize a linkage of primal scene fantasies to self-experiences of instinctual overstimulation. The unseen dimension of biophysiological demand is then included within the realm of self-experience, where the second task of achieving sublimation and secondary autonomy can be negotiated. The obsessive negotiates the first task with great difficulty but not the second. Genitally determined primal scene fantasies of anal penetration establish a structure that is highly defended and traumatic. Concomitantly, incestuous fantasies of anal-genital subjugation and control are structurally linked to the impressions of an overstimulating genital object to form a new boundary for the unconscious system. This union mobilizes defensive activity and is excessively predominant. Although the unseen dimension of instinctual demand is included within the self-system, it is so highly defended that it is inaccessible to processes of sublimation and secondary autonomy. The fixation point on the introjective arm of perception must be defensively maintained and, in conjunction with the reinforcement of reaction formations, prevents any significant degree of integration. The obsessive is dominated by fantasies of anal-genital control of the object to prevent the emergence of genital fantasies of anal penetration.

In the male, a negative oedipal constellation is a partial and pathological solution to the inordinate demand associated with a positive oedipal conflict. The male obsessive perceives feminine qualities as a source of identifications, which aid in the step of structuralizing primal scene fantasies. The attachment to the primary maternal figure is not that strong, and the hunger for closeness to a female can be eased through including feminine attributes within self-experience. The penis is retained as the symbolic organ of attachment to an object, but the influence of anality allows it to be relinquished and received through the route of anal penetration. In the female, a negative oedipal constellation is defensively avoided. In health, a negative oedipal situation serves as a transitional developmental step prior to the displacement of genital interest to the male. The female obsessive finds it intolerable to seek the primary maternal object as a source of genital gratification. The ensuing disappointment is too extreme as a result of the excess of aggression already present, and a displacement of anal-genital interest to the male occurs rapidly. The obsessive female perceives masculine qualities as a source of identification to attain the power of anal control.

The regression of the obsessive is to a remembered position, in which the good self's bad instinctual qualities were not perceived. The structure of the ego ideal is weakened, and the changes that have occurred with the elaboration of the anal-genital fantasies of the oedipal conflict are perceived from this regressive position. This necessitates that symptomatic compromises be formed to attain a measure of stability and regulation and to alleviate the threat of fragmentation. The presence of an open system of perception allows new experiences to be registered, and interactions are sought that reinforce available defensive structures or provide the control weakened by regression. Obsessive symptoms can be ideational, rituals of behavior, or involve compulsive actions. The symptoms remain in the ideational realm when they are successful in regulating instinctual activity but fluctuate in accordance with their degree of effectiveness.

Depression in the Obsessive

Depression is based upon an internal loss. The particular form of a depression is determined by the manner in which the loss is perceived and the specific nature of that loss. In hysteria, depression expresses the loss of contact with the representation of an overstimulating instinctual object (the portal of entry of instinctual demand). The hysteric loses contact with this vitalizing force in the personality and perceives it as the loss of an exciting instinctual object. In obsessional pathology, there is often an ongoing inner sense of an anaclitic loss that influences all perceptual experience. This is related to, and is a reflection of, the excessive frustration that has dominated the early period of development. In addition, there are more acute episodes of depression reflecting the response to a loss of the perceptual focus upon good instinctual self-experiences of mastery and control. The autonomous ego functions are overdeveloped to compensate for deficiencies and highlight these good instinctual experiences. Anal-sadistic drives threaten to emerge, mobilizing reaction formations created by identifications with an anal-sadistic aggressor. This defensive reaction results in a loss of contact with the highly overvalued representations of good self-experience. The aggressive drives pushing for perceptual attention and expression are not well regulated, and the potential for self-destructive thoughts and actions can become acute. During a depressive episode, perceptual attention is occupied with reaction formations of disgust, shame, or guilt, and the function of self-observation becomes harsh and punitive. The depth of the depression depends upon the extent to which the sadistic impressions of an object have been modulated. The more archaic the sadism, the more disgust is manifested. When perceptual attention can be focused upon the representations of good self-experience, effectively reinforced by the background presence of reaction formations and fixed character attitudes, the depression is alleviated.

CHAPTER 7

Obsessive Character Pathology and Obsessive Symptom Formation
Clinical Material

Clinical Material

D was a 35-year-old male who was upset and distraught over two aspects of his life. He was involved in a love relationship, informed that he was too cold, uncaring, and indecisive, and was given an ultimatum that he either get help or the relationship would end. The other concern referred to work. He had periodic episodes of losing control of his anger, was worried about its effect upon others, and suffered greatly from a feeling of guilt. When they occurred, he would go over them endlessly in his mind until they could be rationalized. He repeated each step of his actions until he could somehow assure himself he had done right.

D presented himself as being totally in charge of his behavior. He communicated a sense of desperateness and then immediately shifted to diminishing the intensity of his concern. In the beginning sessions, *D* engaged in repetitive inner dialogues and arguments with the therapist. He took both sides as the therapist was silent. *D* offered interpretations to himself in the name of the therapist and then argued as to their meaning. He frequently began a session with a statement such as, ''I was thinking about what you said about my competitiveness.'' He then reflected upon the truth of the statement and immediately refuted it. He was really a thoughtful, considerate person and not competitive at all. The therapist was silent as *D* continued. He used historical events to back up one argument or the other. For example, he described interactions with three older brothers. These could be seen as competitive, but he was really trying to stand up for his rights when they tried to dominate him. *D* then expressed a vivid fantasy that the therapist was a priest disguised as a psychoanalyst. The therapist's intent was to unearth *D*'s darkest sexual secrets and expose his badness. As he described this fantasy, it evoked a soft laugh within the therapist. The following session occurred shortly afterward.

D entered, carrying a cup of coffee. He set the coffee on a table, lay on the couch, and began to talk about the coffee. It was early in the morning, he was having coffee, and he had thought about the therapist. He felt concern for the therapist's having to come to work early and imagined that he would appreciate having coffee. He wanted to be thoughtful and consider the therapist's feelings. *D* then reflected upon the therapist's silence and wondered if he was appreciative and did not know how to thank him. The therapist stated, "At the moment, all I can see is that you want to put something into me, but I don't know yet what it is." *D* fell silent and recalled his fantasy of the therapist as a priest. He recalled feeling hurt when he sensed the therapist's laugh. Later, *D*'s feeling changed. At first he felt that the therapist was mocking him and then realized that the therapist was laughing at the absurdity of the idea. *D* felt it gave him perspective and made him realize how terrified he was of exposing his sexuality even to himself. He sensed, as he spoke, that he was trying to expose something to himself that frightened him. His words were interspersed with references to the therapist's silence. "That reminds me; I had a dream last night. It's not clear, but a bunch of people were accusing me of being a woman. Why don't you talk?" *D* paused and recalled being fat as a child. He was teased and ridiculed by others, felt effeminate, and wondered if he was homosexual. "I don't know what to make of all this—why don't you say something? Your silence is making me feel mad and frustrated. Isn't there something you can say?" The therapist remarked that he saw his silence was attacking to *D*, but he was not clear yet as to what he needed to hear. *D* began to talk about his responses to silence. Whenever it was silent, he could feel something build in intensity inside of himself. He just wanted the therapist to talk. It felt like the words would ease this inner sensation. That is why he liked to remember the therapist's laugh. It gave him some perspective. *D* became silent and then stated, "I just remembered what I really thought when I bought the coffee. I thought, that son of a bitch will go to sleep on me. I better get him some coffee to wake him up. I better give him this to make him more alive."

E was a very bright and verbal 7-year-old boy. He was described as an ideal child during his first 6 years: neat, orderly, and conforming. He was the only male grandchild and "the apple of his grandparents' eyes." At the age of 6½, both grandparents died within a short period of time. *E* then appeared fearful, developed a series of bedtime rituals, and demanded that the family participate in them. He had to follow a set sequence. If interrupted, it precipitated a temper tantrum or panic attack. His rituals were expanding, and the family, particularly the father, was feeling like a hostage to his emotional well-being. In addition, he could not tolerate his parents' leaving for an evening and began to experience school difficulties for the first time. He could not complete easy reading assignments, would labor for hours on a simple task, and then tear it up in frustration at the slightest mistake.

E began psychotherapy and found it difficult to talk. He sat immobilized in one place, was compliant, and appeared eager to please. He was curious about himself and puzzled about his reactions. In the early months, he described his symptoms and was puzzled as to why he felt so overwhelmed. His symptoms increased in severity, and he did worse in school; this was a profound blow to him. He became more hesitant, fearful, and unable to communicate verbally in his sessions. He appeared frustrated by this inability to talk and saw it as a task he could not live up to. He did not ask questions or seem to expect anything from the therapist. Slowly, he revealed that he had been holding back important information. However, he felt so guilty that he just could not say it. It had been on his mind from the first day. He finally mustered up courage and, with great difficulty, began to describe the deaths and funerals of his grandparents. Everyone around him had been devastated by their deaths, whereas he had felt very little. He masked his inner feeling and pretended sadness. The funerals were exciting to him because there was activity and people that he found very stimulating. It was not until after these events that he began to feel scared and guilty. The following session took place shortly after this revelation.

E began by talking rapidly and without hesitancy. All he could think about was numbers. He counted everything he saw, and he had to end on a number that matched the number of members in his family. If he stopped at 3 he feared a disaster would occur; if he stopped at 5, he was terrified that he would be all alone. He had to stop at 4 or 8 or 12. He was preoccupied with numbers and could not concentrate on anything else. He also was unable to read at school. He constantly anticipated that the next word would make him think of something awful. He had become fearful of tests because he had to read. If he was asked the questions, it did not frighten him. He just could not tolerate reading. At home, he was also becoming more fearful. He had to check the oven to see if the gas was off and then had to go back because he might have accidentally turned it on. When he got into bed, he had to be careful not to touch the bare parts of his body. He had various rituals to cleanse himself and then had to be careful not to contaminate himself by touching. If he touched an exposed part, he had to wash his hands. He did not know what was happening to him. His hands were red from washing so much. However, he had found a way to go to sleep and did not know if he could reveal it. He stopped, started, hesitated, repeated his concern about saying it out loud, paused, and plunged on. ''I have this fantasy that I am the president. I've been afraid to tell you, cause if I say it out loud the president will be assassinated.'' He wanted to bring it out in the open but was now afraid that the president would be shot. The therapist stated he thought E was fearful of the sexual feelings that his symptoms were both hiding and expressing and fearful that the therapist's recognition would shoot down the fantasy that protected him. E became silent and then talked about a friend he had invited to sleep over. They had gotten involved in sexual play by touching each other. It wa extremely exciting, but he wondered if he was a homosexual. He fantasied himself growing up to be a politician and feared that this childhood event would be exposed, publicly humiliating him. The therapist remarked that he thought E was telling him about the guilt associated with his sexual arousal. E responded, ''Oh, I forgot to tell you. One of the things

I worry about is the faucet dripping. By the way, do you have a faucet in here?''

E's response made the therapist aware of his own feeling of excitement at the change in *E*'s ability to communicate. When *E* spoke of the leaking faucet, the therapist wondered if *E* was unconsciously perceiving it. When he then asked about the faucet, the therapist realized that the memory of sexual play was a derivative expressing his experience in the therapeutic relationship. The therapist then referred to *E*'s sensing the therapist's excitement over the way he was talking, which seemed to make him fear that the therapist was getting excited by his sexual fantasies and would be unable to contain it. *E* immediately stated that the faucet that leaked in his house was in the bathroom. He frequently went to check it and noticed his mother undressing in the bedroom as he passed. "Oh, I almost forgot, my father asked me if he could talk to you." He proceeded to describe his father's anger at being enslaved by *E* and his anger that *E* controlled the house by controlling his mother. *E* said, with relief, that he knew the therapist would not talk to his father. It felt good to be able to say "no" to his father.

Discussion

Overideational activities of rationalization, intellectualization, and doing and undoing were clearly evident in both patients. *D* felt great pressure to undo and rationalize the periodic eruption of sadistic impulses. *E* was in a constant state of rumination. *D*'s attempt to adapt to the upsurge of instinctual activity through intellectual mastery was expressed in his repetitive inner dialogue with the therapist. *E* displayed his use of the thinking process in an effort to master instinctual demand, by the formation of compulsive, ideational symptoms. Aggressive and poorly fused libidinal demands were expressed in the compromises of his symptoms, that is, the fear of destroying his family and the sexual overtones in his fear of reading (the next word he read might be overstimulating).

The particular composition of pathological structures is more amply revealed in response to empathic lapses, which require a form of adaptation evocative of their functioning. An unconsciously empathic environment facilitates the ascendency of healthy processes, and, though these pathological structures are still present, they are not as evident. *E* responded to the interpretation of his fear of exposure of his sexual feelings with a memory of sexual play with a friend. The therapist initially heard this as a validation of his interpretation. In the background, the therapist was becoming aware of his own excitement at the change in *E*'s ability to communicate. When *E* associated to the leaking faucet, the background of excitement came to the forefront of the therapist's mind. *E* had unconsciously perceived the excitement and was expressing anxiety that the therapist could not contain it. The acknowledgment of *E*'s unconscious perception and the interpretation that he feared the therapist was sexually excited by his inner revelations evoked an image in *E* of a sexually provocative maternal figure and an enraged father. *E* felt contained and could allow the perception of a woman as a genital sexual object, which immediately elicited the prohibitive presence of the father. The therapist's recognition of his unconscious perception had made *E* feel effective and reminded him of asserting himself with the father.

D illustrated the functioning of an individual with obsessive character pathology. This interaction took place in the midst of the therapist's struggle to grasp the significance of his laughter and highlights the obsessive's characteristic manner of adapting to an empathic lapse. A major difficulty in the treatment of obsessive character pathology is evidenced in this vignette. *D* initially felt hurt in sensing the laugh but then stated that he recognized the therapist was laughing at the absurdity of the idea and not mocking him as he had feared. *D* stressed that the therapist's laughter had given him perspective, made him aware of his fear of exposing sexual secrets to himself, and made him feel better. However, the therapist was aware that, in making *D* feel better, he was colluding with a pathological defense. *D*'s emphasis on rational, logical thinking, and readiness to rationalize an affective experience was clearly reenforcing his characteristic manner of avoiding inner conflict. An effective intervention would have led to the imagery of a healthy interaction and to the revelation of previously repressed instinctual derivatives. In its stead, there was a focus upon conscious mentation. *D* consciously accepted the therapist's collusion with his pathological defenses, yet unconsciously was attempting to call it to attention. His action of bringing coffee was a derivative expressing an unconscious perception of the therapist's "sleepiness." It also represented an attempt to draw the therapist into colluding further in the reenforcement of his defense. The therapist recognized the fact of the collusion but had not yet seen enough of his own motives to be able to interpret effectively and remained largely silent. Ultimately, the therapist became aware of his laughter as a defensive reaction to *D*'s intense negative oedipal homosexual transference. The therapist was unconsciously defusing the intensity by laughter.

D expressed a negative oedipal attachment in his image of the therapist as a priest's seeking his sexual secrets, in his associations to a feminine appearance, and in the dreams in which he is accused of being a woman. *E* also revealed a negative oedipal constellation in his homosexual play, in his fantasy of being exposed as a homosexual, and in his sensitivity to the therapist's excitement. A negative oedipal configuration is a defensive position adopted by the obsessive male when confronted with the enormous castrative threat associated with a genital attachment to a woman. It is a pathological solution to the inordinate conflict engendered by anally influenced, genitally determined instinctual attachments to an object. The overabundance of aggression, associated with attachments to a woman, necessitates a defensive displacement to the male. Some authors, such as Blos (1979), have portrayed the negative oedipal situation as a healthy developmental step in the male. A negative oedipal attachment demands that the original libidinal object be displaced, and the degree of distortion involved in this defensive maneuver is so extensive that it is hard to visualize it as a healthy function. The obsessive's early development is characterized by an overabundance of frustration and an overemphasis on anality; this influences all further phallic and genital instinctual expansion. Women are perceived by the obsessive male as extremely dangerous, and the emerging oedipal conflict necessistates a shift of instinctual interest to the less threatening male object. The negative oedipal situation in a female is the natural progression of a consolidation of the component instincts into a genital drive and is a step toward the developmental task of effecting a displacement to the male. In the female obsessive, a negative oedipal attachment is defensively avoided.

The difference between obsessive character pathology and symptom formation was portrayed by *E* in his description of not being able to read. He could not tolerate the stimulus of reading and the chain of associations it evoked within him. However, he could be read to; that is, the introjective arm of perceptions was open, and he could take in an interpretive statement. He was most fearful of his own regressive process. *D* exhibited the fixed attitudes of obsessive character pathology and, by contrast, could read; that is, the fixation point on the introjective arm of perception was defensively maintained, and he interpreted all incoming stimuli in accordance with their influence on him. He was most fearful of the therapist's reading. *D*'s approach was to exert pressure upon the therapist to reinforce pathological defenses and the anally determined fixation points that supported them. *E* seemingly looked to the therapist for nothing and expected to do everything for himself. *D* and *E* were both expressing the obsessive's need to control. The difference was created by the presence, or absence, of a fixed character attitude. *D* sought an attachment motivated by the need for reenforcement of his defensive attitude. *E* was fearful of the rage and frustration associated with an attachment. In obsessive character pathology, stability and regulation are provided by anally derived fixation points at the foundation of fixed character attitudes. In obsessive symptom formation, there has been a regressive breakdown in function of the fixation point on the introjective arm of perception, and regulation is then provided by symptomatic compromises. This was clearly demonstrated in *E*, who regulated instinctual activity with the entire hierarchy of obsessive symptoms. These ranged from compulsive counting and intrusive ideation to behavioral rituals and compulsive hand washing. His one containing and comforting fantasy involved being president, in which he was omnipotent and in total control. He could not state this out loud without arousing anxiety because allowing the experience of an attachment mobilized the fear of losing control. *E* could not tolerate the perception of his sadistic impulses, which were all embodied in his symptoms, *D* maintained a fixed character attitude and was capable of perceiving these sadistic qualities. He described his mounting frustration in response to silence and could feel the anxiety associated with his limited ability to manage its effects. He sought the therapist's words to diminish the mounting intensity and reinforce his fixed anal character attitudes. *D* was constantly doing and undoing a hostile thought or act. *E*, in adapting to this overloading of aggression, had become passive and compliant. During his early childhood years, he had sustained a fixed obsessive character attitude and appeared to be an ideal child. The eruption of his sadism in response to the excitement of his grandparent's funerals instigated a regression and initiated the emergence of symptoms.

The system of self-representations is constructed similarly in the obsessive with character pathology and with symptom formation. An overloading of aggression reaches its peak during the anal phase and influences all further representation of instinctual experience. Anal qualities of mastery and control dominate within good self-experience and sadistic qualities within bad self-experience. Excessive sensory stimulation in all areas other than the libidinal has led to a hypertrophy in the representation of autonomous ego functioning and a relative diminution in the representation of sensory deprivation and reactions to impingement. There is little available in the self-system to defend against overstimulation. The obsessive utilizes compensatory overelaborations in the object system of representation, and the overdeveloped autonomous ego functions, in the service of defense. Both *D* and *E* consistently displayed this pattern in their mental productions.

Feelings of guilt were a constant inner presence in *D* and *E*; this reflected the effects of an identification with the impinging impressions of an object mobilized in response to the poorly regulated state of sadistic aggression. This prohibitive superego response was harsh, anally sadistic, remained fixed at an early level of organization, and acted in opposition to *D* and *E*'s ego interests. Any expression of instinctual activity was accompanied by the anticipation of a sadistic attack and a compulsive need to undo the powerful feeling of guilt. This was an integral aspect of *E*'s symptoms and of *D*'s feeling attacked by the therapist's silence when his frustration mounted. Anally determined reaction formations, based upon these identifications with a sadistic aggressor, were actively invoked to focus perceptual attention on good self-experience. They were both overly neat, orderly, conforming in their behavior, and worked hard so as not to be seen as aggressive or competitive. *D* was always thoughtful, considerate, and nonaggressive; *E*, was an ideal child.

The line of continuity of prohibitive experience extends from the optimally frustrating impressions of a good object to the impinging impressions of a bad object. The qualities of an object that are admired and selected for identification are primarily those needed for the regulation of instinctual self-experience. In obsessive pathology, the need for a prohibitive force is so great that the sadistic impinging qualities of an anally determined bad object are included within self-experience. The memory traces of an infantile attachment to a good object with bad anal qualities are at the foundation of the fixation point on the projective arm of perception, which motivates the obsessive to evoke these qualities in an external object for the reinforcement of its defensive function. The effect of the therapist's laughter upon *D* was to recreate a mocking, sadistic aggressor, which reinforced this fixation point and mobilized a conscious rationalization as to its helpfulness.

The obsessive has negotiated separation–individuation prematurely and balanced the vulnerability of separateness by participating in the fantasied omnipotence of an object. The resulting structure—the grandiose self—diminishes the accessibility of good instinctual self-experiences. These experiences of mastery and control are involved in a fantasy and are unavailable for adaptive functions, and they disrupt the tenuous balance with inadequately regulated anal sadistic drives. *E*'s fantasy of being president was based on his participation in the object's omnipotence and appeased the extreme vulnerability of being separate. The fear that, in revealing his fantasy, the president would be assassinated reflected the instability of this differentiating structure and the readiness with which aggression could get out of control.

With the structuralization of the ego ideal, perceptual attention is focused upon self-experience. The resulting awareness of the line of continuity of instinctual experience and the recognition of the good self's bad qualities form a fixation point on the introjective arm of perception. In health, this takes place late in the phallic period, has the effect of providing the necessary stability for the structure of castration anxiety to consolidate, and enables the genital fantasies of the oedipal conflict to flourish. This is a transient fixation limiting the influx of new experiences, while the oedipal conflict structures a foundation for object-related perceptions. The resolution of the oedipal conflict is associated with the integration and dissolution of this fixation point, and new object-related experiences can be registered. In the obsessive, the fixation point on the introjective arm of perception is formed prematurely during the anal period, is based on the memory traces of anal-sadistic experience, influences the structure of castration anxiety and the oedipal conflict, and is maintained to defend againt the threat of object-related experiences. Both *D* and *E* exhibited character traits indicative of these fixed, anally determined perceptions. In *E* there was a breakdown in function of the fixation point on the introjective arm of perception at age 7, and *D*'s character pathology continued to be manifested into adulthood.

In health, the fixation point on the projective arm of perception is formed by the memory traces of an infantile attachment to a good object with well-modulated bad anal qualities. There is sufficient flexibility to expand this fixation point by including the impressions of an object with each advancing stage in psychosexual development. The influence of these narcissistic attachments is diminished through the process of depersonification and is eventually replaced with the representations of new and independent objects. The fixation point on the introjective arm of perception is integrated and relinquished with the resolution of the oedipal conflict, and self-expansion no longer depends upon the love of the object but is enhanced through the ability to love an object. The vulnerability to narcissistic injuries is thereby diminished. These advanced steps of development are deficient in the obsessive, and the represenations of the object are overelaborated in an effort to compensate for these deficiencies. This was exemplified in *D*'s fantasy of the therapist as a priest and in his response to the therapist's defensive lapse in empathy. Although he initially felt narcissistically injured by the therapist's laugh, he focused his attention upon extensive speculations as to the therapist's motive. These ranged from visualizing it as a sadistic attack to seeing it as a friendly response to an absurd idea.

The individual with character pathology can only perceive an interaction under the influence of the memory traces of infantile experiences that maintain the fixation points. Verbal interpretations alone are relatively ineffective until the infantile attachments have undergone some measure of replacement. In the early phases of treatment, the obsessive with character pathology recreates interactions that are resonant with the structural makeup of the ego ideal. Sadistic qualities are either provoked or anticipated in the relationship that are a reflection of these infantile attachments that must be replaced. It may be difficult to tolerate the pressure exerted to become sadistic or to have therapeutic interventions be experienced as sadistic. However, it is important to facilitate their expression without participating in their reinforcement. *D* exerted pressure upon the therapist in accordance with the demands of his character. The task was to respond to the pressure by maintaining the framework of the therapy and to offer an interpretation of the unconscious motives expressed in the behavior. The therapist had deviated and was working to reestablish the framework. When obsessive symptoms are in evidence, the introjective arm of perception is open and interpretive interventions are more readily internalized. With *E*, the therapist had deviated slightly, rectified the deviation, and was able to offer an effective interpretation. The therapist must strive to present the combined qualities of a good object. These include those of optimal gratification expressed through well-timed interpretations, silences, and a well-contained framework; of optimal frustration expressed through abstaining from participating in the reinforcement of pathological defenses; and those of a transitional object expressed through facilitating the unfolding of the transference without interference.

Behavior as a Reflection of Character: A Comparison with Hysteria

An individual's behavior is the product of a complex interplay of forces mediated by the personality and expressed in action. A given segment of behavior taken alone cannot reveal the various components that have determined it, but certain behaviors can be expected to result from a particular line of development. Specific qualities of behavior can be anticipated in the developing hysteric and obsessive, although they are in no way restricted to a given diagnostic category. It is mentioned to emphasize that lines of development have behavioral manifestations and to give a sketchy indication of what can be expected and is often observed.

The child prone to hysteria will tend to be whiny, clinging, easily humiliated, overly aware of bodily processes, filled with physical complaints, and imaginative. The developing obsessive child will appear to be self-reliant, contained, preoccupied with order and cleanliness, and less able to be imaginative. The hysterical child is somewhat more resourceful and capable, though appearing less so. The obsessive child appears more integrated, yet is having more serious difficulty. The childhood of the potential obsessive often appears to be progressing effectively until the demands of pubescence emerge. The increased intensity of instinctual demand places an inordinate degree of stress upon the anally determined fixation points that are at the foundation of fixed character attitudes.

In pubescence, the obsessive individual is depressed, preoccupied, and may exhibit transient episodes of symptom formation. The hysteric, who appears troubled in early childhood and through the latency period, seems to intermittently flourish during pubescence. The effort to replace the attachments to primary infantile objects is reflected in a readiness to experience ''crushes.'' The excitement of a new attachment is accompanied by a temporary relief from the overstimulation associated with infantile objects. It is brief, transient, and repeated.

Hysterical and obsessive pathologies may become evident during, and beyond, the period of latency. However, symptoms and noticeable character pathology often do not emerge until triggered by an adaptive demand or an overstimulating event in adolescence or adulthood. The underlying foundation for the development of pathology may be manifested in behavior, before the distortions expressed in symptom or character disturbances have been fully organized.

The Structure of Thought in the Obsessive

Two statements will be presented—one from the beginning of a session and one later in the same session. The first statement is based upon representations of the self and object that are characteristic of the defensive organization in the obsessive. The second statement is indicative of a change resulting from the effects of a therapeutic interaction. The statements are presented in isolation with all significant elements omitted and are explored for their structural composition.

''Am I feeling guilty, or is it because I feel I ought to.''

The idea portrays the self in a relationship with an object, in which a demand is being made that has impinging qualities. The impingement is relatively well modulated with no indication of any ineffectiveness in managing instinctual activity and no hint of threat or danger. The nature of the impingement does not possess the devouring qualities of orality, the humiliating qualities of phallic impressions, or the castrating qualities of a genitally determined object. It appears to represent the subtly sadistic, guilt-producing influence of an anally impinging object. This speculation implies that the statement is founded upon an identification with an anally derived aggressor, which is an important structural determinant of obsessive pathology. The obsessive's tendency to overdevelop the thinking process is hinted at by the intellectualization and rationalization of the feeling of guilt. It appears that an anally determined reaction formation has been mobilized in response to instinctual activity as a manifestation of obsessive character pathology.

The second thought was expressed later in the same session. ''It's very hard for me to tell you that I masturbate. I don't know if it's because I'm embarrassed, or guilty, or because you will tell me I shouldn't do that. It will mess up my sex life.''

The statement is indicative of a change that has taken place in the experience of instinctual activity. The self is represented as involved with a genital instinctual experience and the object as possessing anal, phallic, and genital qualities of impingements. In the first statement, a modulated impinging sadistic object was portraying a well-defended individual with obsessive character pathology. The second thought represents a bad impinging object's invoking guilt, embarrassment, or genitally threatening criticism, and the instinctual activity is libidinal in nature. This suggests that the tenacious attachment to memory traces of anally determined infantile experience has been modified, allowing progressive advancement in instinctual representation.

The fixed perceptions of obsessive character pathology can be modified by replacing the representations of anally derived primary infantile attachments. The impressions of an object comprising the structure of the ego ideal are most accessible and are replaced by a process of identification. This is a gradual process in which a new interaction, parallel with, and evocative of, the origional attachments, is exposed to the integrative forces in the personality through the therapeutic interventions of the therapist. The infantile representation is of a sadistic, impinging object, and the task of effecting a therapeutic influence upon the character pathology of the obsessive may involve an attack. The therapist's interventions are geared to the derivatives expressing unconscious communications, and the patient's defensive avoidance is under attack. These interactions resonate with the representations of infantile attachments to an object and are perceived as a sadistic impingement. The therapist must not only interpret the unconscious motive for this defensive stance, but also acknowledge the attacking qualities that are often present in these interpretive efforts.

CHAPTER 8

The Narcissistically Determined Object-Related Disorders: The Phobias

Pregenital Determinants

Introduction

A *phobia* refers to the avoidance of any stimulus that can evoke anxiety of panic proportions, expressing a threat to the integrity of the self. The anxiety does not have a signaling function as is present with the structure of castration anxiety. It is also not equivalent to the anxiety accompanying a state of overstimulation, which is associated with and bound by proliferative fantasy activity. The anxiety is of a loss of organization and of the functional capacities of the self. This phobic anxiety is at the foundation of all neurotic, object-related symptom and character pathologies. However, in the neuroses, there are structures, mechanisms, and processes available to form the various distortions manifested in pathology.

In the neurotic disorders, cohesiveness and stability are sufficiently structuralized that the genital fantasies of the oedipal conflict can exert their organizing influence. New structures are created enabling the unseen dimension on the continuum of biophysiologic demand and the independent qualities of an object to be registered and represented. The linkages provided by the oedipal fantasies are necessary to structure a foundation for negotiating the shift from a narcissistic to an object-related perspective. In hysteria, these object-related perceptions are partially enhancing and partially traumatic, and the self-system of representations is overdeveloped in the service of defense. The formation of hysterical symptoms signifies that some partial resolution of the oedipal conflict has been attained and that new object-related experiences can be registered with the regulatory support of symptomatic compromises. Hysterical character pathology is manifested when symptoms are ineffective, or when fixed phallically determined prohibitive attitudes are necessary to defend against phallic and genital instinctual overstimulation. Object-related perceptions are traumatic in obsessive forms of pathologies, and the object system of representations is defensively overelaborated. Obsessive character pathology is manifested by fixed anally determined prohibitive attitudes, which are necessary to defend against anal-sadistic and anally influenced genital instinctual demands. Obsessive symptoms develop as a regulatory measure when there is a regressive breakdown in function of the fixation point on the introjective arm of perception.

The formation of a symptom involves a compromise that encompasses the representation of instinctual activity and defense, a superego response, and an aspect that is adaptive to the demands of the external world. The compromises necessary to construct a symptom depend upon the evolution of a considerable degree of representational capacity and structural development. In a phobic situation, this is not the case. A phobia is a narcissistic disorder in which any stimulus that evokes a threat to cohesiveness must be avoided. Although symptoms develop upon the foundation of a threat to cohesiveness, this phobic situation is a precursor of, and motive for, the mental activity that eventuates in forming a symptom. The phobias are the result of an inability to negotiate the shift from narcissism to object relatedness and are fixated to a greater or lesser degree in this perceptual and structural position.

I have referred to the phobias as narcissistically determined and as object-related disorders. They are characterized by a structural organization in which cohesiveness has been established, but the structures uniting and differentiating the self- and object representational systems are highly unstable, function ineffectively, and are threatened with dissolution. The continuing expansion of the component instincts operates as a constant threat to this limited ability to sustain a cohesive state. Tentative and transient advancements in instinctual representation, along with their fantasy elaborations, may provide a skeletal framework for the initiation of an oedipal constellation. However, the instability of the differentiating structures makes the increase in instinctual demand associated with a genital consolidation and elaboration of an oedipal conflict a source of extreme trauma. The particular phobias that are manifested are expressive of the manner in which this underlying psychic organization is perceived.

A given individual may exhibit an object phobia, a self-phobia, or a combined self- and object phobia, and most frequently shifts and fluctuates from one to the other. Each phobia reflects the perception of a bad object's influence, of bad self-experience, or of both, and the fluctuations are based on the unstable functioning of the differentiating structures supporting self-observation. In the object phobias, the structures maintaining cohesiveness are threatened by the effects of recognizing the impressions of a bad object. The threat is symbolized within the self-system of representations directing attention away from this phobic perception because the bad object's differentiating influence must be retained. In the self-phobias, cohesiveness is threatened by the effects of recognizing the bad instinctual qualities of self-experience. The threat is symbolized within the object system of representations directing attention away from a phobic perception of instinctual overstimulation. In the combined self- and object phobias, cohesiveness is threatened by the effects of recognizing bad qualities in both the self and the object, and the threat cannot be psychically elaborated or symbolized. The fixation points that anchor cohesiveness and object constancy are based upon a phobic perception and avoidance, and the phobias are expressed as vague, ominous threats to the self and are often focused upon environmental stimuli.

This formulation is in contrast to the concept of phobias as a symptomatic compromise. A compromise implies that a particular instinct is being granted expression and that it is based upon a specific intrapsychic conflict. It includes an instinctual body ego experience at its foundation that has been represented and expressed in a defensively disguised form and is accompanied by a superego response. Phobias simply symbolize the nature of the threat that must be avoided. Object phobias are represented as a monstrous object threatening the integrity of the self and reflect a high level of instability at the fixation point on the projective arm of perception. Self-phobias are represented as the self's being enclosed, threatened, entrapped, and paralyzed, and reflect the instability having shifted to becoming greater at the fixation point on the introjective arm of perception. The combined self- and object phobias are not represented but are experienced as vague, ominous, poorly defined threats most often attached to environmental stimuli. They reflect the instability of both fixation points and are indicative of a regressive, narcissistic fixation. The choice of a phobic object or situation is determined by its evocative connection to the original infantile experience upon which a phobic attitude has been founded, and the particular phobic position that is manifested depends upon the nature of the stimulus at a given moment. With the phobias, evidence of intrapsychic conflict is minimal and is most frequently postulated by the observer's inference, whereas a psychological symptom contains ample evidence of instinctual activity and defense.

The description of the disorder as phobic and narcissistically determined has reference to the composition of the fixation points, the structures of the grandiose self and ego ideal, and the manner in which they affect perceptual functions. The addition of the term *object related* has reference to the influence of these narcissistic fixations upon the repetitive effort to attain a genital consolidation and elaboration of an oedipal conflict. An object-related orientation is not fully negotiated, although there is a continuing movement in that direction. On the occasions that an oedipal conflict evolves, it is highly unstable, tenuous, easily disrupted, and is characterized by its narcissistic qualities. The unseen aspects of instinctual demand, and of an external object, remain too traumatic to be included within representation. These independent stimuli are perceived as a phobic presence and must be avoided. The need for internal regulation from external objects is perpetuated by the instability of the fixation points and an inability to utilize the prohibitive influences of an object as a regulatory force. These are the individuals Kohut (1971) described as cohesive narcissistic personality disorders, and the narcissistic transferences that they form lead to the formulation of a separate line of narcissistic development.

The agoraphobic individual manifests the presence of a combined self- and object phobia on the verge of a loss of cohesiveness. The need is to be surrounded by stimuli that are totally familiar, as the slightest degree of unfamiliarity is fragmenting in its effects. It is seen in the borderline personality at transient moments when cohesiveness is tenuously established. This discussion will focus upon the cohesive narcissistic disorders in which the thrust of development is toward object relatedness. The first section delineates the early conditions that have determined the structural organization of the personality, the significance this has for further developmental progression, and the nature of its influence upon perceptual functions.

Early Influences in the Development of the Phobias

The discovery of a separate good object's influence connects the self- and object systems of representation, initiates cohesiveness, and expands the boundaries of the self. Object constancy is anchored by the recognition of the good object's bad prohibitive qualities; this is essential for furthering advances in differentiation. The precursors to this crucial developmental step take place within a symbiosis and are a vital factor in determining how it is negotiated. The representations of good self-experience must be sufficiently structuralized at the interior to buffer the disruptive impact of biophysiological demands before they can rise to the surface of the personality to engage in a search for the impressions of a good object. The representations of bad self-experience can then be drawn to the interior of the personality, leaving the structured remnants of reactions to impingement at the surface where they serve a differentiating and protective function. The boundaries of the self are expanded by the perceptual activity of moving around the reactions to impingement in order to locate the representation of a separate good object. A focused area of perceptual functioning (the eye of consciousness) and two arms of perception are established. One, the introjective arm of perception, is an extension of the self-system of representations. The second, the projective arm of perception, effects a connection to the object system of representations. It is through a recognitiion of the good object's bad qualities that a fixation point is established on the projective arm of perception, and the particular nature of those bad qualities has an effect upon its stability.

In the earliest phases of the phobic individual's development, good self-experience has been sufficiently structuralized for the process of separation–individuation to be initiated. At this critical phase, there is a sudden and extreme alteration in the empathic responsiveness of the primary nurturing figure. The developing infant has had a relatively effective period of symbiosis, representations of good self-experience and of a good object's influence are fairly well consolidated, and the first movements toward differentiation are evolving. At this juncture, narcissistic injuries and the reactions to them abound. The originally empathic external object has become impinging in response to the developmental thrust toward separateness. The reaction of the infant is to recognize the absence of a good object in the external world and to engage in a premature search for the influences of a good object in the internal world. The ongoing interaction with an external object has undergone an abrupt change, and body ego experiences of narcissistic injury are registered. In health, the ongoing presence of empathic responsiveness serves as a background to absorb the inevitable narcissistic injuries that result from transient episodes of a lack of empathy. These momentary impingements and deprivations are not out of proportion and act as a spur to the utilization of internal resources, solidifying the separation–individuation process. In this situation, the external object is a source of injury, and the earlier representations of a good object are sought to escape that injury. The process of separation–individuation is instigated defensively, as a consequence of trauma, prematurely during the oral period.

The events occurring during the later phases of orality are creating an unstable foundation for the establishment of cohesiveness and for the manner in which the lines of continuity of prohibitive and instinctual experiences are perceived. The early oral phase has provided an abundance in the representation of good self-experience and a good object's influence; this is reminiscent of what has transpired in health and to some extent in hysterical forms of pathologies. In the hysteric, libidinal overinvolvement has been sustained over an extended period of time. However, in the phobic disorders, there is a sudden change in the qualities of empathy specifically with the ascendency of a movement toward individuation. The shift takes the form of impinging attacks upon autonomous functioning, which interfere with the progression that has been gradually emerging. These are not the impingements of libidinal overinvolvement seen in the developing hysteric, and although excessive frustration is suddenly created, it is not equivalent to the ongoing level of frustration that is a part of the obsessive's early development. These are direct impacting, unempathic attacks that impinge with each thrust for individuation. They may result from any set of conditions that ruptures the existent empathic environment such as bodily illnesses or the birth of a sibling, although most frequently, they involve the emotional attitude of the primary nurturing figure. The mother is often extremely narcissistically oriented and remarkably sensitive and responsive within a psychological symbiosis. The infant, in emerging from the symbiotic interaction, stimulates this narcissistic nurturer to react with rage at the loss of a needed external source of supply, and the infant's budding individuality is attacked. The suddenness, intensity, and nature of the narcissistic injury is responded to by engaging in an internally directed search for a separate good object's influence. The subsequent formation of a fixation point on the projective arm of perception takes place prematurely during the oral period. The abrupt alteration in a relatively adequate unfolding of advancing sequences in development presents a difficult task, and the structures that eventuates are highly unstable and limited in their effectiveness. The combination of a period of libidinal involvement shifting to excessive frustration is at the foundation of the mixture of hysterical and obsessive features that characterize these narcissistically determined, object-related disorders.

The response of searching for the representation of a good object is an expression of autonomy and individuality. The fusion and merger experiences, which are essential for establishing a foundation upon which separation–individuation can be initiated, have been sufficiently consolidated at the interior for this process to continue. However, they exert a strong regressive pull, especially with the impact of narcissistic injuries, which presents a threat to the tenuous progression toward separation. The anxiety of a loss of separateness is an additional impetus for furthering the process of individuation. The impressions of a good object that are perceived are those of an orally gratifying object elaborated into a fantasy of an all-giving nurturer. The good object's bad prohibitive qualities are also orally determined and are represented as devouring and incorporative. The fixation point on the projective arm of perception, designed to maintain differentiation and anchor object constancy, is based upon a recognition of these bad oral qualities and is highly unstable. This is in contrast to the firmness of this point of fixation when it is established at later developmental periods. The instability is partly due to the degree of perceptual maturation and partly due to the nature of the bad object that is perceived. The immaturity of perceptual functions diminishes the capacity for differentiation, and the resultant fluctuating object impressions tend to blur the distinction between an all-gratifying good object (evocative of a loss of differentiation) and an incorporative bad object. These orally derived representations of attachment to an object have a powerful influence upon perceptual processes; this is accentuated by the overloading of orally determined self-experiences of aggression. The threat of loss of differentiation has spurred the premature search for the impressions of a separate good object's influence, and the awareness of the good object's incorporative qualities establishes differentiation on the basis of a phobic perception.

The sudden influx of narcissistic injuries at the onset of individuation intensifies the pull toward lack of differentiation. Autonomous functioning is operative under an excessive degree of stress, and each advance increases the anxiety of its loss. During moments of stress, or periods of overstimulation, cohesiveness, may be ruptured. The result is in transient episodes of being drawn into the poorly differentiated perceptual positions of fusion and merger. These moments are generally transient, and cohesiveness is readily reestablished by evoking the representations of a good object through contact with a transitional object or an empathically responsive external object. The phobias are narcissistic disorders in which cohesiveness has been established and progression toward object relatedness is manifested. The developmental task of shifting from a narcissistic to an object-related orientation has not been negotiated.

The Grandiose Self and Ego Ideal in the Phobic

The location of a separate good object's influence and the formation of a fixation point on the projective arm of perception connect the self- and object systems of representation, expand the boundaries of the self, and establish a more advanced level of psychic organization based on cohesiveness. In the phobic disorders, this developmental step is negotiated but is tenuous and very unstable. In addition, the recognition of separateness is associated with an exaggerated experience of vulnerability and helplessness that is of traumatic proportions. The grandiose self is structured to balance that experience by utilizing the orally determined fantasy elaborations of an optimally gratifying object. With stage and phase specificity, the experience of vulnerability is tempered by the linking fantasy of an anally derived omnipotent object, which maintains cohesiveness on a firmer basis. This grandiose self, based on the fantasy of an all-giving orally gratifying nurturer, is an unstable structure. It is vulnerable to the threat of loss of cohesiveness from the influences of orally incorporative impressions of a bad object and does not offer a firm enough foundation to support continuing instinctual expansion.

In forming the grandiose self, the representations of good oral instinctual self-experience are structurally linked in participation in a fantasy, and the self-system is threatened with fragmentation from the intensity of poorly fused oral aggressive instinctual demands. In conjunction with the unsteadiness with which cohesiveness is being maintained, there is an urgent motive to strengthen the bonds uniting and differentiating the two systems of representations, by including within self-experience those influences of an object that can alleviate the stress. The ego ideal is then structured prematurely, under potentially traumatic conditions, late in the oral phase when perceptual processes are relatively immature. The ego ideal is formed by a process of selective identification, in which the autonomous ego functions are elaborated into fantasies of self-potentials and linked to admired and needed qualities of an object. The greater the degree of perceptual maturity, and the more the representations of the object are well modulated and differentiated, the more identifications are discriminating and selective. The qualities of an object that are most admired are those that best compensate for deficiencies or that provide what is most immediately needed. In this situation, although the regulation of instinctual activity is sorely deficient and the prohibitive influences of an object are desperately needed, the impressions of a bad object are too threatening and must be avoided. The developing phobic individual utilizes the best alternatives, which are the representations of an orally determined optimally gratifying object. The need for instinctual regulation must be obtained from interactions with external objects, reflecting the evolving inability to consolidate an effective independent superego agency.

The ego ideal is structurally linked to the representation of an optimally gratifying oral object, whereas the grandiose self makes use of the fantasy elaboration of that same aspect of an object's influence. The composition of these two unifying and differentiating structures is in close approximation, and the contiguity operates to create the fluctuations in perceptual attention that characterize the shifts from one phobic experience to another. When these two structures are formed in a stage- and phase-specific manner, they are composed of differing facets of an object's influence and are uniquely adapted to regulate the perceptual functions in the conscious and preconscious systems. They then insure cohesiveness, offer the means for increasing stability and regulation, support instinctual expansion, and provide a foundation for increasingly discriminating perceptual functions. In the phobic disorders, the grandiose self and ego ideal are functionally operative as a unit, fluctuate in their regulation of perceptual functions, and maintain cohesiveness with a level of instability that offers only limited support for instinctual expansion.

The prohibitive influences of an object possess oral incorporative qualities, are threatening to cohesiveness, and are phobically avoided. The process of identification with an aggressor is inaccessible, so that reaction formations cannot be established. The gradation of instinctual experience, in not being clearly demarcated, remains as an ongoing source of overstimulation. The increase in instinctual activity associated with the evolution of the component instincts and their consolidation into a genital drive is an overwhelming threat. Although there may be some transient forays into an orally influenced genital consolidation, the demands of an oedipal conflict are so highly traumtic that an immediate and rapid regression is initiated. In these narcissistically determined object-related disorders, unseen aspects of experience are phobically avoided because they evoke the threat of narcissistic injury or of oral incorporation. The anticipation of narcissistic injury emanates from the mental impressions of the trauma of early development. The anticipation of oral incorporation is a reflection of the pull toward fusion and merger that remains as an active force in the personality. Any progression toward elaborating the genital fantasies of an oedipal conflict invokes a threat to cohesiveness, with regulatory structures that are deficient and ineffective. The only available response is a regressive retreat to the relatively more stable, orally determined, narcissistic fixations.

The heavy infiltration of narcissistic injuries at the critical point of early individuation has created defensive and compensatory responses that affect perceptual functions and distort the representation of incoming stimuli. The fixation point on the projective arm of perception is based on a phobic perception of the good object's bad qualities and is readily threatened with dissolution. The grandiose self and ego ideal are structured to maintain cohesiveness and provide a foundation for continuing developmental progression. These unifying and differentiating structures are composed of the same aspect of an object's influence, which places cohesiveness on an unstable basis. This is reflected in the fluid shifts and fluctuations that take place, in which compensatory distortions are emphasized in the object system of representations, alternating with defensive distortions in the self-system of representations. When the object system is accentuated, obsessive features are manifested, and when the self-system is emphasized, hysterical features are in evidence. The combination of hysteric and obsessive configurations in the same individual is a characteristic of these disorders. It is necessary to shore up whatever defenses are available at a given moment, as cohesiveness is threatened by both the influences of a bad object and increases in instinctual activity.

Separation–Individuation, Cohesiveness, and the Formation of Differentiating Structures

A state of cohesiveness is manifested by a well-defined system of self- and object representations that are united and differentiated. It signifies that the process of separation–individuation has been negotiated by the formation of mental structures designed to connect the two systems in a way that facilitates continuing self-expansion. The grandiose self and ego ideal are the major structures whose functions direct the course of attaining advancing levels of psychic organization. The particular composition of these structures, and hence the functions they serve, is determined by the nature of self-experience and of an object's influence that has been represented. The grandiose self is based upon an instinctual attachment to the fantasy of an optimally gratifying object, establishes an internally directed perceptual boundary for the superego and regulates the mental activity of the preconscious system. The ego ideal is based upon an identification with the impressions of an object that are most needed, is more affected by external reality, establishes an externally directed perceptual boundary for the superego, and is ideally suited to regulate the mental activity of the conscious system.

In healthy development, the ongoing empathic responsiveness of an external object acts as a background to absorb the effects of the inevitable narcissistic injuries, lapses in empathy, and separations that are an integral part of human existence. These inevitable occurrences then serve as a stimulus to further the process of individuation and to stimulate the use of functions that strengthen self-experience. The representations of impingement and deprivation that result are in a balanced proportion and are a necessary component for the regulatory and defensive structures required to further the thrust of progressive development. In the phobic individual, when the individuating process has attained sufficient dominance to allow emergence from the lack of differentiation embodied in a symbiosis, there is a marked change in the empathic conditions of the surrounding environment. The primary nurturing object has become a source of narcissistic injury, which prematurely instigates a search for the represented influences of a separate good object. The process of separation–individuation is initiated defensively, in the absence of a buffer for modulating narcissistic injuries. The recognition of separateness is associated with an exaggerated experience of vulnerability and helplessness, at a time when perceptual and regulatory functions are immature. There are some individuals with a structural organization similar to the phobic disorders that have a different developmental history. They have had a faulty representation of the background object of primary identification and an unusually sensitive and empathic environment. The responsiveness of the environment has successfully mitigated the effects of this deficiency, which eventuates in a tenuously held cohesive organization. The difference is in the absence of fluctuations from one phobic position to another and the presence of an unstable field on which mental impressions are represented. The instability that charcterizes the phobic disorders is manifested in rapidly fluctuating mood swings, shifts in levels of self-esteem, and fluid changes in the degree of anxiety and the nature of what is threatening. These rapid shifts and changes cannot occur in the genital character or in the object-related disorders due to the functioning of the grandiose self and the ego ideal. The ego ideal, in particular, maintains a firm connection to the influences of an object that can regulate and stabilize self-experience.

Mental structures are formed by the linking function of fantasies, which connects the representations of self-experience to the impressions of an object. Those structures that involve an attachment to an object are instinctual in nature and are linked by a fantasy of the object. Those structures that include the impressions of an object within self-experience are based on identifications and are linked by a fantasy of self-experience. The autonomous ego functions are the only aspect of self-experience capable of effecting an identification because the use of perception is required to determine the varied qualities of an object that are needed. The experience of vulnerability associated with separateness motivates the formation of an instinctual structure—the grandiose self. With stage and phase specificity, anal experiences of mastery and control are linked to a fantasy of the good object's omnipotence, which balances the vulnerability. I have called it "the grandiose self" because it involves participation in a fantasy and depletes the availability of good instinctual self-experience. The resulting imbalance increases the threat of overstimulation and motivates the formation of a new and separate structure—the ego ideal. This structure is formed by a process of selective identification. The impressions of an object that are needed, admired, and included within self-experience are those that are most effective in strengthening the capacity to manage instinctual activity. The processes involved in separation–individuation are the same for all individuals; it is the conditions under which it takes place and the composition of the self- and object representational systems that create the differences.

In the phobic individual, a premature process of separation–individuation has been negotiated under conditions that exaggerate the vulnerability experienced with separateness. These conditions include the absence of empathic responsiveness, the presence of impingements, and the immaturity of perceptual functions. Early representations of orally determined experience are almost exclusively utilized to structure the grandiose self and ego ideal. The fantasy of an all-giving nurturer, elaborated from the impression of an optimally gratifying good object, provides the link for the grandiose self. The impressions of an optimally gratifying object are included within self-experience to form the ego ideal. The optimally gratifying impression of a good object, which formed prior to the trauma, has been utilized in uniting and differentiating the self- and object systems of representations. The grandiose self and ego ideal are thereby interconnected in their functioning; there is a limited degree of discrimination between them; and cohesiveness is maintained by structures in which fluctuation can occur with little opposition.

The body ego experiences and object impressions of the original trauma create a heightened sensitivity to lapses in empathy. The effects of even transient empathic failures are manifested by a rapid regressive shift in perceptual attitude. In the object-related disorders, narcissistic injuries have an effect but do not instigate such a massive alteration in psychic organization. The underlying unifying and differentiating structures of the grandiose self and ego ideal develop as separate entities, are more distinct in their areas of function, and provide more regulation and stability. In addition, the line of continuity of prohibitive experience is a pathway for including the restraining forces of an object within self-experience. In the phobic disorders, the optimally frustrating impressions of an object are too evocative of ongoing narcissistic injuries, and the line of continuity of prohibitive experience is a pathway to the phobically avoided, orally incorporative impressions of a bad object. The optimally gratifying influences of a good object, which have been missed with the onset of trauma, are most needed. The ego ideal is then structured with the same aspect of an object's influence as the grandiose self, and their functions operate in concert with each other.

The Effect of the Absence of Reaction Formations

Reaction formations are an effective regulator of instinctual activity. They are based upon the process of identification with an aggressor, in which the prohibitive influences of an object are included within self-experience. In health, they are stage and phase specific and are utilized only at transient moments of stress or overstimulation. In the object-related disorders, reaction formations are an integral part of the fixed character attitudes designed to regulate instinctual overstimulation. The stability of the fixation point on the introjective arm of perception is reinforced by their availability.

In the phobic disorders, the distinction between an all-giving nurturer and an incorporative object is somewhat blurred; fusion–merger experiences continue to be active forces within the personality; the prohibitive influences of a bad object are phobically avoided; and the process of identification with an aggressor is unavailable. The absence of reaction formations does not clearly delineate the transition of instinctual experience from good to bad qualities, and, as a result, the fixation point on the introjective arm of perception is relatively unstable. However, the structuralization of the ego ideal has included the influences of a good object within self-experience, making it possible to symbolize the phobic threat to cohesiveness. The degree of stability within the self-system of representations will determine the degree to which the component instincts can expand and reflects the movement toward object relatedness.

The Composition of the Self- and Object Representational Systems in the Phobias

The representation of good instinctual self-experiences reflect the abundance of phase-specific instinctual gratification that transpired during the early oral phase. However, instinctual experiences that do not require defense are markedly diminished in the later phases of orality, in proportion to the change in the empathic conditions of optimal gratification. Good instinctual self-experience is sparcely represented from this point through the advancing stages of psychosexual development. All adaptive demands or intrapsychic processes that invoke the activity of this facet of self-experience will display a strong early oral influence. The autonomous ego functions are hypertrophied, reflecting the extent to which they have been utilized in the premature search for a separate good object's influence. The background object of primary identification is solidly represented, which is manifested in the degree of containment that is present in an empathic environment. The impact of narcissistic injuries, which has profoundly affected the course of development, has distorted but not interfered with the process of individuation, due to the firmness of this representation. The background necessary for well-defined self- and object systems of representations to be united and differentiated depends upon the degree of its intactness. There are some individuals who have attained cohesiveness with a background object of primary identification that is defective. Although empathic contact with external objects is inadequately represented or represented as injurious, a high level of empathic responsiveness to this inner instability has resulted in a sufficiency of good qualities of experience for some degree of cohesiveness to evolve. The instability would be evident in the disturbed sense of containment, even in the presence of an empathic environment.

Bad instinctual self-experiences are vastly enlarged during the later oral period, which affects all further instinctual expansion. The overloading of oral aggression, represented as envy and greed, colors the way body ego experiences associated with anal, phallic, and genital sensations are registered and represented. Reactions to impingement, which are heavily represented in the later oral period, are utilized as a major defensive response to any increase in instinctual demand. The fantasies of fight, flight, and withdrawal are linked to the impressions of an impinging object to form a boundary delineating the transition from unconscious to preconscious mental activity. It is a rigid, inflexible boundary leaving little leeway for the formation of instinctual derivatives. The representation of sensory deprivation increases dramatically as development proceeds beyond the adequate period of a psychological symbiosis. Fantasies of emptiness are elaborated that serve as a defensive response to instinctual overstimulation.

The optimally gratifying impressions of a good object that have formed during the early oral period are quite extensive. It is this aspect that is sought in the premature movement toward separation and individuation, and the fantasy elaboration of an all-giving nurturer is incorporated in the structure of the grandiose self. The optimally frustrating impressions of a good object are minimally represented in the early phase and, with little gradation, merge into the impingements of an orally incorporative bad object. This abrupt transition contributes to the degree of instability of the fixation point on the projective arm of perception. The lack of gradation in the line of continuity of prohibitive experience, in conjunction with a premature onset of separation–individuation, when perceptual functions are immature and fusion–merger experiences an active force, results in an inadequate distinction between the qualities of an all-giving mother and those of an orally incorporative bad object. These factors are at the foundation of the phobic attitude toward the influence of a bad object. The impressions of a transitional object are particularly important because the thrust for individuation occurs with an overdetermined need for contact with the influences of a good object in the presence of forces that jeopardize it. Engagement with and dependence upon transitional objects in the external world are exaggerated. They have the effect of amplifying the representations of a good object, modulating the instability of the grandiose self and ego ideal, and alleviating the acuity of phobic anxiety.

The instinctual aspect of a bad object is predominantly orally determined, although anal, phallic and genital qualities may be included in a limited fashion. The primal scene fantasies that are elaborated are a source of extreme trauma and must be warded off or phobically avoided. The impinging impressions of a bad object, reflecting the narcissistic injuries of the later oral period, are predominant and elaborated into fantasies of oral incorporation.

The process of identification with an aggressor, which at later stages of development is effective as a regulatory, prohibitive force, is largely inaccessible because the influences of an orally incorporative object are too threatening to the already tenuous state of cohesiveness. The impressions of a depriving object are both plentiful and readily available to form defensive alignments with self-experiences of sensory deprivation.

The Fixation Points and Their Relationship to Phobic Symptoms

The fixation point on the projective arm of perception is based on a recognition of the good object's bad oral incorporative qualities. The lack of a clear distinction between the anxiety of lack of differentiation evoked by the impressions of a good object and the threat of dissolution evoked by the influences of a bad object make this fixation point extremely unstable. Differentiation is founded upon a phobic attitude, in which the effects of a bad object threaten cohesiveness and must be avoided. The degree of instability cannot support compensatory elaborations in the object system of representations because any significant amount of psychic activity threatens the capacity to maintain this fixation point.

The premature structuralization of the ego ideal late in the oral period is associated with a recognition of the good self's bad oral instinctual qualities. A fixation point is thereby established on the introjective arm of perception with an inability to clearly demarcate the transition from good to bad instinctual self-experiences. This fixation point, although unstable, due to the absence of a well-defined distinction between good and bad instinctual qualities, has a greater capacity to support the psychic activity of symbolization and derivative formation within the self-system of representations.

The initial threat to cohesiveness is present within the system of object representations due to the nature of a bad object's influence. The tenuous fixation point on the projective arm of perception, which must be maintained to anchor object constancy and differentiation, acts as a stimulus to the representational capacities of the self-system. The fixation point on the introjective arm of perception has sufficient stability to allow the psychic activities of symbolization and derivative formation, and the threat to cohesiveness is symbolically represented as an object phobia. The elaboration of psychic content within the self-system of representations alleviates the stress on the vulnerable fixation point on the projective arm of perception; all stimuli that resonate with the influences of a bad object are avoided; and there is an excessive dependence upon external objects to provide internal regulation. The degree of stability may enable instinctual representation to include anal, phallic, and, to some extent genital components. The anlage of an emerging oedipal conflict, with its increase in instinctual activity, is inordinately traumatic. The fixation point on the introjective arm of perception is in danger of dissolution from the effects of instinctual overstimulation, and the threat to cohesiveness has shifted to the self-system of representations. A rapid regressive shift transpires, in which the vulnerable fixation point on the introjective arm of perception is maintained by a phobic attitude toward bad instinctual self-experiences. The fixation point on the projective arm of perception, having been eased of undue stress, has a limited ability to support the elaboration of psychic content in the object system of representations, and a self-phobia is symbolically represented. The self-phobia is often a transient phase as the regression continues to the position of a combined self- and object phobia. The fixation points on both the projective and introjective arms of perception are tenuously maintained, and there is very little capacity for symbolic representation. In this narcissistic fixation, cohesiveness is threatened by instinctual overstimulation within the self-system and by the influences of a bad object within the object system.

A unique characteristic of these narcissistically determined, object-related disorders is the ability to elaborate psychic content in the self-system with an absence of activity in the object system and for the same individual to fluctuate and elaborate psychic content in the object system with an absence of activity in the self-system. The interrelated functioning of the grandiose self and ego ideal facilitates these ready shifts from one system of representations to the other, which is a consequence of their having formed from the same aspect of an object's influence. The ego ideal utilizes the optimally gratifying impressions of a good object, and the grandiose self utilizes its fantasy elaboration of an all-giving nurturer. This is the underlying foundation for the coexistence of mixed hysterical and obsessive pathological constructions.

An object phobia manifests progression toward the evolution of object relatedness. However, the demands of an oedipal conflict are totally overwhelming and instigate a regressive shift to a self-phobia or to a combination self- and object phobia. External objects are depended upon as a source of regulation, and lapses in empathy or even short separations reactivate early traumata and can be excessively disruptive. The combination self- and object phobias are a final attempt at narcissistically fixating the state of cohesiveness, although a given individual will most frequently shift from one phobic position to another.

The unstable fixation point on the introjective arm of perception and the absence of reaction formations amplify the sensitivity to unconscious perceptions of the qualities present in an interaction. These narcissistically determined and object-related disorders are extremely perceptive of, and vulnerable to, narcissistic injuries. This is in contrast to the object-related disorders, in which the defensive organization is capable of absorbing the narcissistic injuries resulting from momentary or transient lapses in empathy. The object phobia is a symbol of the threat to cohesiveness that is invoked when the influences of a bad object are activated. Empathically responsive interpretations of unconscious communications are evocative of the representations of a good object; their stabilizing presence eliminates a phobic situation; and the therapist is experienced as an instinctual object. When the therapist is experienced as a phobic object, it is indicative that the unconscious perception of unempathic qualities in an interaction is being expressed.

CHAPTER 9

The Narcissistically Determined Object-Related Disorders: The Phobias

The Significance of the Oedipal Situation

Introduction: The Conditions Necessary for a Shift from Narcissism to Object Relatedness

A narcissistic orientation is necessary to gain sufficient structuralization within the personality so as to continue self-expansion from a separated, individuated, and autonomous position. This is accomplished through the vehicle of an oedipal conflict, which enables the representation of the unseen dimension on the continuum of biophysiological demand and the independent qualities of an external object. The formation and resolution of the oedipal conflict result in a new level of psychic organization, which is characterized by the ability to further growth from the effects of object-related rather than narcissistic experiences. In order to negotiate this shift, cohesiveness must be established on a solid foundation, object constancy firmly anchored, the regulatory influences of an object fairly well consolidated and available, and the disruptive effect of new stimuli under control. This means that the grandiose self and ego ideal must function effectively in uniting and differentiating the self- and object systems of representations; the fixation points on the projective and introjective arms of perception must add their stabilizing function; and castration anxiety must be consolidated into a signaling and regulatory structure. The stage is then set for the expansion of instinctual activity that gives depth and body to the enlarging complexity of human experience. In this well-structured psychological setting, the genital fantasy elaborations of the oedipal conflict can flourish and exert their organizing influence.

The genital fantasies of the oedipal conflict provide the necessary linkages for structuring a new boundary of the unconscious system of mental activity and a well-regulated pathway of instinctual integration. The representations of narcissistically determined experience can then either occupy a place in the id of the dynamic unconscious or be utilized in forming derivatives in the preconscious system. Incestuous fantasies reflect the defensive, regulatory activity of the unconscious boundary and are in a balanced proportion with the primal scene fantasies reflecting the movement of the instinctual demand toward integration and secondary autonomy. Cohesiveness is secured at the interior of the personality, and an uninterupted flow of instinctual activity provides the impetus for continuing growth and expansion. These new structures are at the foundation of the capacity to recognize and register the unseen qualities of an object and provide the wherewithal to sustain an object-related perspective. In health, an object-related perspective is enhancing, whereas in the object-related disorders, it is potentially traumatic and defended against to varying degrees.

The Preconditions for Object Relatedness in the Phobias

The dramatic change in quality of the phobic individual's period of symbiosis results in an overvaluation of good self-experience and a good object's influence. The sudden shift from an empathic surrounding to unempathic impingements has initiated a premature process of separation–individuation. The earlier representations of fusion and merger continue to operate as an active force, exerting a regressive pull to a lack of differentiation. In health and in the object-related disorders, these fusion and merger experiences have become structuralized as a foundation for absorbing narcissistic injuries; this is manifested in a basic sense of the goodness of the self and object. In health, and to a lesser extent in the object-related disorders, ongoing empathically responsive interactions are present as the infant emerges from the lack of differentiation of a psychological symbiosis. The body ego experiences and object impressions of these empathic interactions are registered and represented, enabling firm structure building to occur in a stage- and phase-specific manner. The developing phobic individual does not have a foundation for absorbing narcissistic injuries and has to depend almost solely upon the representations of what was an adequate symbiosis to structuralize cohesiveness. Although cohesiveness is established, the structures that maintain it are extremely unstable and continuously threatened with dissolution.

The impressions of a separate good object's influence, which, in being recognized, form the first bonds of cohesiveness, are orally determined. The awareness of the good object's bad oral qualities anchors object constancy by forming a fixation point on the projective arm of perception, which is based on orally incorporative impingements. There is a similarity between a bad orally incorporative object and the regressive pull exerted by fusion–merger experiences because fusion and merger involve a lack of differentiation and have the characteristic of being swallowed up. Perceptual functions are immature, the capacity for making fine distinctions is limited, and the transitions from good qualities to bad qualities are poorly distinguished. The differentiating influences of an object are threatening to differentiation, arouse anxiety of panic proportions, and must be avoided. The fixation point on the projective arm of perception is thereby based upon a phobic attitude toward attachment to an object. The fantasy of an all-giving nurturer, the effects of fusion and merger, and the incorporative impingements of a bad object are fine and important distinctions that are difficult to make with an immature perceptual apparatus. The fixation point on the projective arm of perception is designed to stabilize cohesiveness by making this distinction and is very vulnerable to a loss of this function.

The grandiose self and ego ideal are also unstable, are constructed from the same impressions of a good object, and function as a unit. The structuralization of the ego ideal is associated with an awareness of the good self's bad instinctual qualities. This also transpires prematurely, late in the oral period, when orally sadistic experiences of greed and envy are at their height. The fixation point formed on the introjective arm of perception has a relatively greater degree of stability, from the influences of a good object that have been included within self-experience. The stress upon cohesiveness exerted by the influences of a bad object is somewhat alleviated, facilitating the expansion of the component instincts toward consolidation into a genital drive.

Instinctual expansion exhibits a strong oral coloration and extends the aleady limited capacity for regulation. The beginning forays into representing phallic and genital instinctual experiences are accompanied by an emerging state of trauma, and an attempt to consolidate the lines of continuity of prohibitive and instinctual experiences into the regulatory structure of castration anxiety. In health and in the object-related disorders, castration anxiety is a stable union of instinctual and prohibitive forces that serves a signaling and regulatory function. It is an essential condition for genital instinctual activity to be adequately represented and reinforces the stability of the fixation points. In the phobias, some degree of genital instinctual activity and its associated prohibitive response may be initiated, but the instability of the fixation points prevents the consolidation into a functional structure. The upsurge of instinctual demand poses a threat to cohesiveness within the self-system of representations, as the fixation point on the introjective arm of perception loses its stabilizing function. The prohibitive influences of an object, which have retained their oral incorporative qualities, offer little regulation and must be phobically avoided. Castration anxiety is not capable of organizing into a unified regulatory structure serving a signaling function but is experienced as a trauma instigating a regressive shift to a narcissistic fixation.

An object phobia is the most advanced of the narcissistically determined object-related disorders. The fixation point on the projective arm of perception is tenuous and vulnerable to a loss of its differentiating function. The fixation point on the introjective arm of perception has a degree of stability that allows psychic content to be elaborated within the self-representational system. The threat to cohesiveness is then symbolically represented as a bad object threatening the self. In some individuals, there may be enough stability to support expansion of the component instincts and even a measure of consolidation into an orally influenced genital drive. The object phobia is accompanied by anxiety-laden progressive thrusts toward the formation of an oedipal conflict. This movement toward object relatedness is threatening and usually short lasting. The particular oedipal configurations that are initiated are profoundly affected by the instability of the mental structures maintaining differentiation. In both males and females, the primary nurturing object is inordinately threatening and infused with oral incorporative qualities. In the male, this necessitates a negative oedipal position, whereas the female phobically avoids the developmental step of a negative oedipal constellation. The phobic disorders display the potential of movement toward the formation of an oedipal conflict that is not fully realized. The consolidation of the component instincts into a genital drive requires an enlarging capacity for instinctual representation, and there is insufficient stability and regulation to do so. The phobic individual displays advancements toward object relatedness that cannot be sustained, while continuing to hold a narcissistic perspective upon all experiences. For this reason, the disorder has been described as narcissistically determined and object related.

The Status of Internal Regulation in the Phobias

The grandiose self is linked by the fantasy elaborated from the impressions of an optimally gratifying good object. It is formed during the oral phase, and the fantasy of an all-giving nurturer is evocative of fusion–merger experiences, making it an unstable structure. The ego ideal utilizes the impressions of an optimally gratifying good object (rather than the fantasy elaboration), which forms a more stable structure. They are so closely connected that each responds to the functioning of the other, allowing cohesiveness to be sustained, although on an unstable foundation.

The influence of an orally incorporative bad object exerts a constant threat to maintaining the tenuous fixation point on the projective arm of perception. The process of identification with an aggressor, rather than providing regulation, would intensify the difficulty with differentiation. The prohibitive influences of an object are unavailable, which exaggerates the dependence on external objects for regulation. When cohesiveness is present on a firm foundation, anchored by a fixation point that functions effectively, identifications with an aggressor and the resulting reaction formations act as a powerful restraining force to instinctual overstimulation. Reaction formations create a clear demarcation between good and bad instinctual self-experiences; this operates to strengthen the stabilizing funciton of the fixation points. In the phobias, reaction formations do not develop; the transition from good to bad instinctual self-experience remains as a gradation that can readily become traumatic; and the stability of the fixation point on the introjective arm of perception is weakened.

The ego ideal has strengthened the functional capacities within the self-system of representations and facilitated the formation of symbolic derivatives. These mental activities provide an element of regulation that aids in furthering the representation of the component instincts to the point of their consolidation into a genital drive. That amount of instinctual expansion, with an absence of effective regulatory responses upon an unstable foundation, shifts the major threat to cohesiveness to the fixation point on the introjective arm of perception. The stress in the object system is temporarily alleviated by this shift, and the threat is symbolically represented as a self-phobia. The regression is often a transient step toward a narcissistically fixated, combined self and object phobia. The threat to cohesiveness is then present at both fixation points, and there is little capacity for representation in either the self- or object system.

Within a narcissistically structured personality, when instinctual activity is of an intensity that is impinging, it mobilizes the reactions to impingement and establishes a boundary for the unconscious system. This boundary does not possess the necessary flexibility to foster the formation of instinctual derivatives, which invokes stringent limitations to instinctual representation. In health and in the object-related disorders, the genital fantasies of the oedipal conflict have structured a new boundary for the unconscious system, allowing a greater range of instinctual activity. In addition, a structured pathway for instinctual demands to gain access to sublimation and secondary autonomy has not been established, and all autonomous ego functions are occupied with the defensive task of maintaining cohesiveness.

The Relationship of the Fixation Points
to a Genital Consolidation

The tenuously established fixation points do not provide the level of inner stability necessary for genital fantasies to flourish into a full elaboration of an oedipal conflict. The fixation point on the introjective arm of perception, in functioning ineffectively, continues to register the new stimuli of the external world. During the period of oedipal organization, it is essential for new experiences to be buffered and registered as familiar by the functioning of stabilized fixation points because the influx of new stimuli is too disruptive in its effects. In health, new object-related structures evolve with the oedipal conflict, and its resolution is associated with alterations in the fixation points. A process of depersonification enlarges the fixation point on the projective arm of perception and loosens the tenacious hold of infantile attachments to an object. The fixation point on the introjective arm of perception is relinquished, as instinctual experiences requiring defense are integrated and attain secondary autonomy. These processes are totally unavailable to the phobic individual. The mental structures that formed in response to the trauma of early development are an integral part of the perceptual boundaries of the preconscious and unconscious systems of mental activities, and the inability to absorb narcissistic injuries has left a heightened and reactive sensitivity to any unempathic stimuli. Although a fixation point has formed on the introjective arm of perception, the level of instability leaves it open to the effects of new experiences. The phobic individual is exquisitely and unconsciously sensitive to the barest hints of impingements and is extremely vulnerable to narcissistic injury.

Instinctual self-experiences and the prohibitive influences of an object both pose a threat to cohesiveness, and the mental activity of elaborating fantasies places stress upon the stabilizing function of the fixation points. The combination tends to exaggerate the activity of unconscious perceptions; this is reflected in the derivatives that are evoked by an interaction. Empathically responsive stimuli evoke the representations of good self-experience and of a good object's influence, strengthen cohesiveness, and support movement toward object relatedness. Unempathic stimuli evoke the representations of the original trauma, weaken cohesiveness, and instigate a regression. The fixation point on the introjective arm of perception, in not preventing or buffering the impact of new experiences, increases the reactive sensitivity to narcissistic injury. The dependency on external objects for internal regulation accentuates the effect of lapses in empathy, which create a phobic situation.

Instinctual representation, although poorly regulated, can reach a point of genital consolidation. The increase in instinctual activity alters the point of vulnerability to a loss of cohesiveness. Initially, the influences of a bad object threaten cohesiveness at the fixation point on the projective arm of perception. With the onset of an oedipal conflict, the intensity of instinctual demand threatens cohesiveness at the fixation point on the introjective arm of perception. The response, due to the absence of regulation and stability, is a rapid regressive shift in structural organization. The stress of maintaining a fixation point on the projective arm of perception in the presence of instinctual expansion is momentarily alleviated, which enables the representation of a bad object to be elaborated in fantasy. This regressive movement offers a transient element of regulation; the self is symbolically represented as entrapped; and a self-phobia is manifested. It can only be sustained for a short period of time before the regression continues to a narcissistic fixation with no capacity for symbolic representation. The narcissistically determined, object-related, phobic disorders shift and fluctuate from one phobic position to another, depending upon the internal and external conditions. In an empathic environment, the most advanced levels of organization will be manifested, and in an unempathic environment the most regressed.

The Nature of the Oedipal Conflict

The phobic individual has had sufficient structural development to negotiate separation–individuation, attain cohesiveness, and for repression proper in its earliest stage to emerge as the major defensive activity of the ego. There is a consistent impetus to advance individuation and to move toward object-related experiences. This progression is profoundly affected by the pathological distortions in structure formation that have been an integral aspect of earlier developmental periods. Instinctual experience is inordinately influenced by the predominating effects of orality, and the developmental task of shifting from a narcissistic to an object-related orientation is entered into but not successfully negotiated. The increase in instinctual activity associated with the oedipal conflict is totally overwhelming because the foundation upon which it takes place is so unstable. There may be transient progressions into the initial phases of an oedipal constellation, but they invoke a regressive return to unstable, narcissistically determined phobic fixations. The deficiency in regulatory and stabilizing forces within the personality does not allow the full flowering that is necessary for object-related perceptions to be structured.

Object-related perceptions are an integral aspect of, and the product of, the organizing function of the oedipal conflict. New stuctures are formed that provide the internal capacity to register and represent the unseen dimension on the continuum of bio-physiological demand as well as the independent qualities of an object. The developing phobic individual is in a potential state of trauma as movement occurs toward the formation of an oedipal configuration. The fixation point on the introjective arm of perception is unstable and threatened with a loss of function by the increased intensity of instinctual demand. Castration anxiety has not consolidated into a unified regulating and signaling structure. The ego ideal and grandiose self maintain differentiation on an unstable foundation, and the prohibitive influences of an object are phobically avoided and unavailable. The budding genital fantasies require an immediate defensive displacement from the primary object, which is too threatening and infused with oral incorporative qualities. In the male, the ensuing negative oedipal situation is in itself traumatic and mobilizes a narcissistic regression. In the female, there is a rapid displacement to the male as a genital instinctual object, and the resulting positive oedipal constellation is equally traumatic. In these narcissistically determined, object-related disorders, an oedipal conflict that extends beyond its early and tentative beginnings is a new experience. The male requires a working through of a negative oedipal conflict, and the positive oedipal attachment is a new experience. The female must resolve the defensive aspects of a positive oedipal attachment to engage in the new experience of a negative oedipal conflict. It is only then that a positive oedipal position can be entered as a step toward integration.

The phobic individual is strongly motivated to seek interactions with external objects that will have the effect of strengthening cohesiveness and regulating self-esteem. In a therapeutic environment, unconsciously determined empathic responsiveness communicated by interpretive interventions evoke and amplify the representations of a good object. Under these conditions, it is possible for the furthest level of developmental progression that has been attained to be manifested. An empathic environment elicits the structural organization of an object phobia, and the therapist is experienced as an instinctual object. An unempathic environment elicits the structural organization of a combined self- and object phobia, and the therapist is experienced as a phobic object. Self-phobias reflect the transition from one to the other. In the object phobias, there is sufficient regulation to elaborate psychic content into the formation of symbols and derivatives and for instinctual representation to reach an orally influenced, genital consolidation. It requires the sensitive, unconsciously attuned interpretive activities of a therapist, within a well-managed therapeutic framework, for the oedipal conflict to be fully elaborated. The onset of an oedipal constellation is a repetition, but its flourishing is a new experience. Inevitable empathic lapses and unavoidable separations will continue to trigger regressions to the narcissistically determined phobic attitudes. However, there will be an enlarging ability to absorb the narcissistic injuries they entail and to gradually integrate the abiding effects of the early developmental traumata at their foundation.

The Threat of Loss of Cohesiveness

The fantasy of an all-giving nurturer, the oral incorporative impressions of an impinging object, and the experiences of fusion and merger are in close approximation to each other. In conjunction with the contiguity in function of the grandiose self and ego ideal and the exaggerated dependence upon external objects for regulation, any lapse in empathy can evoke a shift from one to the other. In addition, the instability of the fixation point on the introjective arm of perception heightens the reactive sensitivity to unempathic stimuli. The stress on the fixation points can reach an intensity that eventuates in a loss of their functional capacities, and cohesiveness is then ruptured. It can occur in response to the trauma of instinctual overstimulation or in response to the overriding impact of an orally incorporative object. A momentary and massive regression is instituted, fueled by the regressive pull exerted by fusion and merger experiences, overcoming the ineffective differentiating function of the grandiose self and ego ideal. The distinctions between self and object are lost, as the lack of differentiation associated with fusion and merger is predominant. Cohesiveness is readily reestablished by contact with a transitional object or with an empathic external object. The impressions of a separate good object's influence are amplified; this reinforces the unifying and differentiating structures of the grandiose self and ego ideal. This phenomenon is frequently observed in the initial phases of psychotherapy, when lapses in empathy and separations can be shattering in their effects.

I have referred to these disorders as narcissistically determined, object related, and phobic in nature. They are in a transitional position between narcissism and object relatedness, with a continual striving for progression that eventuates in trauma. The mental structures at the foundation of the personality have been formed as a defensive response to narcissistic injuries, which results in an inability to absorb the inevitable narcissistic injuries of human existence. Even minimal criticisms, lapses of empathy, or separations from a loved object trigger a profound loss of self-esteem and depressive responses, which are aspects of the persistent narcissism. The experiences of self-esteem and mood are largely dependent on the particular qualities of a given immediate interaction. This lability in mood and self-esteem is a source of ongoing concern and reflects the reactive awareness of the underlying instability and dependence upon external objects for regulation. Finally, they are phobic in nature because there is an avoidance of all stimuli that pose a threat to cohesiveness. A phobic situation is at the foundation of all symptom and character disturbances, but in those situations, cohesiveness is secure, and there is a large capacity for instinctual representation and regulation. The one exception is in the severest forms of obsessive symptoms, where the threat to cohesiveness is a factor. In the phobic disorders, the structures at the foundation of cohesiveness are unstable. They are constantly under stress, and the task of maintaining differentiation is inordinately difficult.

Depression in the Phobic Disorders

In health, and in the object-related disorders, representations of empathic contact with an external object during the oral phases of development are structured within the personality and available to buffer the impact of narcissistic injuries. In the phobias, they are utilized to structure differentiation and cohesiveness. The trauma that has affected the course of development is the basis of the internal loss at the foundation of frequent episodes of depression. The grandiose self and ego ideal are composed of structured linkages to the representation of an orally derived, optimally gratifying object. When the functioning of these structures is interfered with by the influences of a bad object or by an overwhelming intensity of instinctual demand, there is a loss of immediate contact with the impression of a separate good object's influence. That loss is evocative of the original trauma, in which there was a loss of contact with an empathically responsive external object. It is a frequent occurrence, is instigated and alleviated readily, and is the internal reenactment of that original trauma.

The dependence upon external objects for regulation is associated with a search for, and sensitivity to, empathic qualities in an interaction. Impingements, separations, and empathic failures elicit recurrent disappointments, and initiate a depressive episode. The movement toward object relatedness is also disruptive to the tenuous contact with the influences of a separate good object and is the frequent source of a depressive response. The depression is alleviated by any experience having the effect of reinforcing the impressions of a good object. These include making contact with an empathically responsive external object, locating a transitional object, or through regressing to a previously held narcissistic fixation.

The Narcissistically Determined Object-Related Disorders: The Phobias
Clinical Examples and Discussion

Introduction

Phobic disorders are manifested as an object phobia, a self-phobia, or a combined self- and object phobia. The pathology of this disorder has resulted from an inability to negotiate the developmental step from narcissism to object relatedness, and the shift from one phobic position to another is the sequela of the manner in which separation–individuation has been negotiated. The grandiose self and ego ideal are structured from the same aspect of an object's influence, which establishes differentiation on an unstable foundation. When these structures are composed of differing aspects of an object's influence, a higher level of stability and differentiation is maintained. This has particular relevance in regard to the ego ideal, which is based upon including within self-experience the specific qualities of an object that are deficient and most needed. The motive for these selective identifications is expressed through the admiration of those qualities. In health, the masculine or feminine qualities that strengthen self-identity and offer effective restraints are most admired. In the hysteric, the need for regulation of phallic instinctual activity makes the optimally frustrating or prohibitive, humiliating qualities of an object most admired. In the obsessive, the need for forceful restraint of anal sadism highlights the sadistic impinging qualities of an object as admirable. In the phobias, the trauma occurring with the onset of differentiation makes the optimally gratifying impressions of an object most needed and admired. The distinction between the structures of the grandiose self and ego ideal are then blurred; their functions are intermingled; and the readiness to alter one phobic attitude with another is a constant presence.

The Object Phobias

The following example is of a young adolescent boy primarily exhibiting the structural organization of an object phobia. The object phobia represents the self as threatened by an object, possessing orally determined qualities that are engulfing and devouring in nature. It symbolizes the threat to cohesiveness at the fixation point on the projective arm of perception. The elaboration of psychic content within the system of object representations and the cognitive functions involved in thinking are curtailed by the instability of this fixation point.

F was a 14-year-old boy referred due to his parents' and school's frustration in knowing how to handle and respond to him. *F* was almost always right and fiercely determined to maintain that position. He refused to do homework in school because no one could provide him with a reason that was sensible to him. In addition, he could prove to the school that the reasoning of their officials was faulty. An authoritative stance would be adopted, and *F* would mock and laugh at this attitude. The school authorities were upset that no consequences seemed to affect *F*. No matter what was tried, *F* simply smiled or laughed. At home, he was in a constant battle with his parents. In their words, he refused to face or accept reality. He had many interests and was involved in numerous projects that required intense concentration and work. However, they all were activities that he enjoyed. He totally refused to extend himself if he was not interested. He was creative and effective in what he did, but only on his own terms. When given some other task, *F* would simply refuse and remain steadfast. There were also episodes of extreme temper outbursts, particularly with his mother or younger brother. These explosive responses were triggered by some injustice and seemed to have a large element of control. His mother felt very guilty, as *F* was frequently accurate in his perceptions. His father was a pragmatic individual who was not concerned with the quality of *F*'s academic performance but was deeply concerned with his inability to live "within the system." *F* was perceived as being spoiled, lazy, undisciplined, living by the dictates of his grandiosity, and unable to adapt to the world of reality. Three previous efforts had been made to seek professional help, with *F*'s refusing to return after one or two sessions. He did not resist going; he only resisted returning after a short trial.

F came willingly to his first appointment as he had done in the past and talked openly of his parents' and school's concern. His descriptions were exactly parallel to those presented by his parents. When *F* saw a reason for doing something, he did so gladly, but no one gave him valid reasons that made sense to him. Further, when he voiced an objection, no one showed him where he was wrong. They only insisted that he do as others did or stated that it was in his best interests. He spoke of his many and varied activities and of his friends. He valued relationships highly, and was deeply concerned with injustices and moral issues.

He had found two people in his life who gave him good reasons for doing things. One was a piano teacher. *F* played piano by ear and was pleased by his ability to play, although everyone was upset because he refused to learn to read music. They saw his talent and were angry with his refusal to develop it. The piano teacher did not try to teach him music but tried to help him develop his own skills. He presented disciplined activities to follow and explained how they could foster his innate potentials. The other was a Hebrew teacher who explained the importance of learning the language. *F* had begun with no intention of learning, but when the teacher talked to him about language as a way of solidifying a union with his forefathers, *F* disciplined himself to do so. This teacher talked about the importance of being a separate individual, and this so impressed *F* that he became involved in learning the new language.

F then asked what the therapist thought about all that he had said. The therapist was aware that *F* had provided him with derivative expressions of how to establish a working relationship.

The therapist stated that *F* had shown qualities within himself that were expressions of his effort to be a separate individual with the strength to stand up for what he believed and to establish his uniqueness. The therapist also heard how important it was that *F* and the therapist see reasons for working together. The therapist wondered if *F*'s questions were expressing a sensitivity to the therapist's feeling that there was a lot left unspoken that would give such a reason. The therapist, in listening to *F*'s desperate fight to maintain his autonomy, separateness, and individuality, was becoming aware of his own unconscious sensitivity to the underlying vulnerabilities that were unspoken. *F* immediately responded by asking, "What do you mean?" The therapist stated that he meant that *F* seemed to be fighting very hard for his autonomy but was not very effective, and the therapist sensed that there were things he hadn't spoken of that hampered him. Further, when *F* told the therapist of his piano and Hebrew teacher, he was describing what he needed from the therapist if they were to work together. *F* stated, "I want you to listen. There are many things I can't talk about. I know this is a place for me to talk, but I won't talk about some things." *F* was adamant in his refusal. The therapist remarked that he thought *F* was talking about what he didn't want to all of the time. The therapist thought *F* was wondering if the therapist would ignore what he heard or would not let *F* know when he heard. Much later, *F* informed the therapist that this moment was when he decided to engage in therapy. He began to feel that he could talk.

In the early months *F* talked about his wide ranging interests. In the course of describing these interests a constant theme inadvertently slipped in. It involved an inner sense of danger, injury, and destruction. When it would "slip" out, *F* made a joke of it. For example, in describing his interest in magic, he would laughingly wonder what someone would do if they were missing a finger; or he wondered how a person with no arms could use a computer. On one occasion he came in tearfully and signaled the therapist to be silent. He went on to say that he could not talk, and wanted the therapist to forget about it. He then joked about how impossible it is to forget something when someone tells you to forget it. He slowly and hesitantly began to reveal his profound phobia. He was terrified when he went to bed each night, feeling that there was something in his closet that would come out to destroy him. He knew it was ridiculous and made no sense. He engaged in various rituals to distract himself. *F* was totally mortified that he was so frightened. He had a great deal of trouble going to sleep, and no one knew of it. He had kept it hidden, feeling it as a sign of weakness. *F* was shocked that he was telling the therapist, and now he did not know what to do about it. It made it no better or no worse. He went on to describe his fears. He had just learned of a beloved grandfather's serious illness. He felt himself becoming terrified about the idea of death, and this had reminded him of his phobia. He had not wanted the therapist to talk so he could bring it up in his own way. He did not want the therapist to elicit it from him.

The following session took place shortly afterward. The therapist had received an upsetting phone call just prior to the session. *F* came in, looked at the therapist, and asked, ''Do you believe in ESP?'' He went on to describe his interest in ESP, telekinesis, reincarnation, and various mystic phenomena. He elaborated upon how careful he had to be as to who he talked to about it: ''People think you are crazy if you believe in these events. Unless they believe in it too, they think of you as strange. If they believe in it, then you can share your ideas and experiences.''

The therapist gradually became aware that he had not processed the previous phone call very well. Its effects had lingered as *F* entered the room. The therapist was still involved with ''the craziness'' of the phone call, and it appeared that *F* had unconsciously perceived it. The therapist stated that he thought *F* sensed some inner disturbance in the therapist and was concerned that it would be projected onto him. *F* became silent and then thought of his piano teacher. This teacher was helpful and encouraged *F* to play well. He returned to his interest in ESP and to the things he sensed in other people. He gave many examples of coincidences that he seemed to anticipate and reflected upon his sensitivity to unconscious messages. *F* looked up at the therapist and asked ''Was there something? Will you tell me?'' The therapist said he thought *F* was checking to see if the therapist was now ready to listen because he had not been at first. *F* became pensive and talked of how preoccupied he had been with his fear of a monster in his closet. He suddenly became aware that what he feared was inside of him, not outside of him. He had been exquisitely sensitive to things in other people, which made him feel that everything he feared was outside of him. That is what confused him about the closet. He knew there was no one there, but the fear was exactly the same as if there was someone there, and he sensed it. It made *F* feel that there was someone hidden, and he was sensing their presence just as he sensed things unseen in other people. He was now aware, both in his sensing things in other people and in his fear of the closet, that it was connecting with something inside of him. He now felt able to think about what he feared. He could look at his own thoughts the same way that he looked at another person when he tried to sense their unconscious messages. He then said, ''There is one thing I've never told you. It looks to everyone like I'm very creative and do a lot. The truth is I never complete anything.'' *F* described coming to the end of any task and suddenly abandoning it. He felt an inner fear and tried to make it look as though he had finished. ''There's something about finishing a job that scares me. When I said that, a song went through my head. I'll bet that's a message from inside of me.'' He paused and remarked that he felt silly and yet knew it was not silly. ''I want to be able to let things come into my mind and think about them.'' *F* puzzled about the song and then recalled that it was titled ''My Life.'' The lines had to do with someone's life being cut off, and the song was bringing him a message that to finish a task was like ending his life. He felt so terrified of his life's ending that he could not complete anything. It was the feeling of something in the closet. *F* stopped and laughed, ''I just had a funny thought. Something in the closet feels like something in my mind I've kept closed off. It's trying to come out and give me a message.''

F reveled in how good it felt to think this way. Previously, he could only be afraid, pull back, avoid thinking, and then feel humiliated about pulling away. *F* felt like something was expanding that allowed him to think. He then recalled his mother's telling him a story that never made sense until just now. His mother told him that as an infant, he was extremely special to her. When he began to assert himself, she became so enraged that she could not tolerate him and beat him. She hated herself and went into treatment. Later, his brother was born, and she involved herself with the brother in a similar way. *F* had reacted to the birth and early infancy of the brother with all of the reactions she thought he had from the first period of trauma. The first instance was at less than a year, the second at age 3. The intensity of his hostility to the mother made her think it was from his period of infancy. What he understood was that, whenever he looked at his brother, he felt like he wanted to hit him in a particular manner. He liked his brother, and it has always puzzled him. He realized that the way he wanted to hit his brother was identical to the way his mother described hitting him. *F* then noted the time ending (uncharacteristic for him) and left.

F was a child with vast potentials, who gave evidence of having had an excellent symbiotic experience that was traumatically ruptured at the point of individuation. His fierce fight to maintain a feeling of separateness and autonomy barely concealed the enormous vulnerability that was constantly present. There was an underlying anticipation of total gratification by an all-giving nurturer, which appeared to balance the extremes of his vulnerability. In addition, his adaptive capacities were strengthened when the qualities he admired in an object were included within his experience. These admired qualities were best expressed in his descriptions of the piano and Hebrew teachers. They involved support and encouragement of autonomy and independence; this appears to have an anal derivation. However, they were not so much in the service of mastery and control as they were empathically responsive to efforts at individuation. The phobic individual's development is characterized by an effective early oral period of symbiosis, which is severely traumatized with the onset of individuation. This was the theme of his mother's story. *F* was very special until he manifested his uniqueness and then was viciously attacked. The effect was to motivate a premature process of separation–individuation. The grandiose self was structured with the fantasy of an orally determined all-giving nurturer to balance the excessive vulnerability of separateness. The ego ideal was structured with impressions of an object that reflected the transition from orality to anality, which was indicative of somewhat greater stability. Kohut (1971), in formulating a separate line of narcissistic development, placed emphasis upon the role of empathic failures in creating self-pathology. The patients he described were diagnosed as narcissistic personality disorders—a category that could be applicable to *F*. *F* displayed an orally determined characterological fixation, with a phobic attitude toward the influences of a bad object.

F had successfully negotiated separation–individuation but had done so prematurely. The grandiose self was structured during the oral period and embodied the representation of good instinctual self-experience's uniting with the fantasy of an all-giving nurturer. *F* perceived himself to be the recipient of everything from the world, only listened to what made sense to him, and was grandiose in his expectations. At the same time, he was depleted in adaptive capacities, unable to realize vast potentials, and sought the influences of an object that could strengthen his ability to function. He did not seek external objects to idealize, but looked for a source of much needed identifications. Idealizations require that the image of an object be filled out, and they are depleting, whereas identifications include qualities of an object within self-experience and are enhancing. *F*'s identifications were based upon the needed optimally gratifying influences of an object that comprised the structure of his ego ideal. This is what *F* found in his teachers and was probing for in the early sessions with the therapist. In the beginning, it was important for *F* to know what the therapist had to contribute; later it became important for the therapist to know *F*.

Cohesiveness is first established with the recognition of the mental impressions of a separate good object. At the outset, differentiation is maintained through the active functioning of perception. With stress or fatigue, there is a return to the lack of differentiation of fusion and merger. The awareness of the good object's bad qualities occurs by registering the impressions created by the line of continuity of prohibitive experience, in which the optimally frustrating influences of a good object shade into the prohibitions and impingements of a bad object. A fixation point is formed on the projective arm of perception, anchoring object constancy and maintaining a constant differentiating influence. In health, this occurs during the anal period when good instinctual self-experiences of mastery and control are in the forefront. The union with anally derived fantasies of an object's omnipotence structures the grandiose self and provides a perfect match to obviate the vulnerability associated with separateness. The resulting depletion motivates the structuralization of the ego ideal, and a pathway is available for including the restraining influences of an object within self-experience. The degree of restraint that is necessary will be in proportion to the amount of regulation that is required. This process of identification with an aggressor is totally unavailable to the phobic individual because the frustrating impressions of an object are too evocative of the early trauma, and orally determined impingements are phobically avoided. The superego remains at an immature level of organization, its prohibitive functions are not effective in regulating instinctual demands, and it cannot function as an independent agency. The dependency upon external objects for regulation is thereby exaggerated. *F* was driven to create interactions, in which prohibitions would be enforced, to attain some measure of regulation. At the same time, he had to include an active effort to asssert his autonomy because he could not allow the experience of dependency. He sought external objects that provided regulation that he could fight against and had to be correct in his battle to deny the importance of the object. Concomitantly, he was hungry for identifications with an autonomous figure, who in no way either engulfed or imposed upon him.

The grandiose self and ego ideal in the object phobia demand constant reinforcement. The instability is a consequence of their having formed with the same aspect of a good object's influence; the grandiose self utilizing the fantasy of an all-giving nurturer and the ego ideal the impressions of optimal gratification. There is sufficient support, particularly from the ego ideal, to enable psychic content to be elaborated within the self-system of representations. In *F*, the content of his phobia was represented as a danger to the self, of destruction by an unseen, devouring monster in his closet. An orally determined impression of an impinging bad object's influence possesses these same qualities, and his phobia symbolized the overwhelming threat to maintaining differentiation. It was constant with the formulation of a fixation point on the projective arm of perception being rigid and unable to expand, so that the bad qualities of an object upon which it is founded place the integrity of the self in jeopardy. This fixation point has depended upon a recognition of bad qualities that are orally engulfing; this is so threatening that they can only be phobically avoided. The threat is then represented within the self-system as an object phobia. *F* had to recognize a bad object's influence in order to maintain differentiation, but these particular qualities were too threatening to perceive, and the phobia was his solution. By way of contrast, the hysteric and obsessive not only recognize the bad qualities of an object to establish differentiation but also utilize them as a source of restraint and prohibition. Through the process of identification with an aggressor, they are perceived, admired, and included within self-experience. *F* was humiliated by an inability to talk about his phobia and took the defensive stance of refusal. He anticipated and feared the therapist would expect him to talk about that which he could not even think about. This defensive posture stabilized cohesiveness in *F* because he depended upon the object phobia to maintain differentiation. With all of his intellectual capacities and vast array of skills, he was incapable of thinking about what threatened him the most. In addition, to complete a task required that he ultimately perceive what was most frightening, and he was immobilized. The best he could do was to represent the threat as an object phobia and avoid any stimulus that resonated with it.

The impetus and motivation for attaining an object-related orientation are created by the need for representing increases in the intensity of instinctual demand. In health, a phobic situation emerges at the point of a shift from narcissism to object relatedness, which activates the full elaboration of an oedipal conflict. A fixation point is maintained on the introjective arm of perception for a transient period of time to provide the necessary stability while new structures insuring object-related perceptions are organized. The narcissistically structured personality severely limits the representation of instinctual activity and is in a phobic situation when confronted with the increase in instinctual demand associated with a genital consolidation of the component instincts. Any developmental progression requires the capacity to register object-related perceptions. *F* indicated the tremendous threat engendered by the structural limitations to instinctual expansion, although he had gained sufficient structuralization to elaborate and symbolize the threat. Phobic symptomatology and a narcissistic orientation to all stimuli were manifestations of the pathological forces that interfered with his functioning. The representations of infantile attachments to an object needed to be replaced in order to alleviate the phobic situation. The hero worship of his admired teachers reflected what was missing and required, as he looked for qualities of uniqueness, discipline, regulation, and autonomy. The relationship with the therapist offered an opportunity for a new object to be represented, so as to be accessible for selective identifications that could support cohesiveness and strengthen the capacity for instinctual expansion. It was essential for the therapeutic interaction to resonate with the infantile representations that were most prominent; this involved those comprising the ego ideal. The impressions of a good object were colored by an enormous need to be as special and unique as he was to his mother during the early oral period. They were also affected by the impressions of the paternal imago, whom he distantly respected and admired. This figure, though readily taking on the dimensions of a phobically avoided bad incorporative object, also was seen as a potential source of restraint. Identifications with the therapist's unconsciously responsive interpretive attitude were initially parallel with these infantile representations. The experience of having his unconscious perceptions validated amplified the representations of a good object's influences; identifications became increasingly independent of their infantile foundations; and the ego ideal functioned more effectively in providing stability and regulation. Projective processes and ideational activity became more functional as the threat to cohesiveness abated. As *F* described it, he could now think. He was able to be introspective, fostered by the stabilized function of self-observation, and his object phobia was no longer in evidence.

In later sessions, *F* displayed a capacity for instinctual representation that encompassed progression through all of the phases of psychosexual development. Instinctual derivatives proliferated without creating a phobic situation. He portrayed the status of orality in describing his effort to lose weight. There was an intense hunger that fueled an enormous appetite, but he felt a sense of mastery in containing and channeling it. Anal qualities extended to his exerting sadistic control over external objects, and there was much conflict associated with sadistic aggression. Phallic configurations were abundant and expressed in a preoccupation with exhibitionistic activities and prohibited voyeuristic temptations. The latter were accompanied by anxiety, reflecting the beginning consolidation of castration anxiety as a signaling and regulatory structure. He had great difficulty in revealing an emerging genital awareness, and a budding oedipal conflict was manifested in derivative associations to being charming to females and working hard to make their male friends jealous. Although these vivid instinctual derivatives were associated with anxiety, there was no longer a phobic response. The shift from narcissism to object relatedness was in the process of being negotiated.

The following session occurred many months later. *F* began talking animatedly about telling several friends that he was in therapy. He recalled an earlier time when he had been fearful that someone would find out and that he would have felt humiliated. Now he valued the experience more, felt comfortable in letting others know, and laughed as he described his discovery that others he had told were also in therapy. He then paused and spoke of his new girlfriend. He met her on a trip and fell deeply in love. She lived far away, which made it extremely painful to be so in love and to be so distant. He talked with her on the phone each week and felt an intense longing afterward. It was like being on a diet and seeing your favorite foods on display, Your appetite was whetted but not fulfilled. He wished he could turn it off because it was so painful. *F* paused and talked more of being intimately connected to his girlfriend. They were able to understand each other without words. The therapist commented that as *F* talked about communicating without words, it appeared to be his way of letting the therapist know that he was talking about the therapist without words. It reminded the therapist of *F*'s earlier fear that he would not be able to allow himself to feel such an intense attachment. *F* looked embarrassed and noted that when he thought of turning it off, he was trying to draw back. He remembered how afraid he had been of feeling love for someone. At the time, he felt he was being strong. Looking back, it seems like he was being defensive and closing himself up. Now he felt open to the experience and wanted to risk it. He sensed that it must have been that way with his mother early in life. He recalled fearing that he would never feel love for someone, and, now though it is difficult, he values it highly. He might get hurt or rejected, but that seems relatively unimportant because being able to love meant everything.

F had begun to experience intense instinctual attachments. He communicated this new development by describing his feeling in telling others of his therapy. He was committed to the relationship and valued it. He then associated to an intense love relationship, which appeared to be a derivative expressing a genital, instinctual attachment to the therapist. This loved figure was far away and, to a large extent, unattainable. Simultaneously, the loved object was connected to him by a bond of empathic resonance that made the distance tolerable. The representations of instinctual attachments that were embedded in the id of his dynamic unconscious exerted an influence on his experience with a loved object, and he feared being hurt and rejected. The shift from a narcissistic orientation associated with infantile objects to an object-related orientation associated with new objects was reflected in the narcissistic concerns of hurt and rejection that were anticipated and in the experience of being enhanced from feeling love for the object. The therapist's interpretation was followed by an expanded awareness of the effects of his developmental experience upon his ability to love and upon his defensive responses.

F's difficulty in regulating instinctual demands was proportional to the level of his narcissistic fixation. There was sufficient stability for a marked increase in instinctual representation to take place and for an oedipal conflict to be elaborated. The consequence was in the newfound capacity for an object-related orientation.

The Self-Phobias

The following example is of a young man primarily exhibiting the structural organization of a self-phobia. The model is of claustrophobia, which reflects the threat to cohesiveness by the effects of instinctual overstimulation. The fixation point on the introjective arm of perception is formed with a recognition of the good selfs' bad instinctual qualities late in the oral period. These bad qualities are of oral greed; they are devouring in nature and influence all further instinctual expansion. The stabilizing function of this fixation point is jeopardized by any significant increase in instinctual activity. In the self-phobias, the threat to cohesiveness has shifted from the influences of a bad object to the immobilizing impact of instinctual demand. The result is in a phobic attitude toward bad instinctual self-experience, symbolically represented as being trapped within a confined space. Psychic content can no longer be elaborated within the self-system of representations, and there is some capacity for psychic activity in the system of object representations.

G was a 17-year-old boy referred to the therapist as a last resort. He had been to three other therapists, of differing orientations, who determined that his phobia was untreatable, and the family doctor had suggested seeing an analyst. G was a very bright, extremely intellectual, and well-groomed young man. He began by speaking of the outrage he felt in not being able to overcome his fear of being in a classroom with other students. He felt helpless, and his inability to go to school had been managed through home teaching. However, he had an acute and pressing problem. He had a scholarship to college, and if he did not take an upcoming test, he would lose it, and he felt desperate. The time was getting closer, and he was totally unable to even think of entering the classroom. G went on to talk about why he is so outraged. He described himself as smart and accustomed to ''commandeering'' the classroom. It came as an enormous surprise to him when his symptom first became manifest. Prior to this, he had reveled in the classroom experience. He now felt as though his whole life was being ruined. When he was younger, he was teased about being a brain and felt like an outcast. As he got older and peers became more mature, he was not teased as much. He felt fortunate that he was also an excellent athlete because this diminished the intensity of the teasing and elaborated on his athletic skills and accomplishments. The worried expression on his face deepened, he paused, and expressed concern that the therapist would misunderstand and perceive him as bragging and arrogant. He was working hard to present an accurate picture of himself, and, to do so, he had to describe his exceptional qualities. He referred to the other therapists he had seen. One attempted to desensitive him from his phobia and was unsuccessful. G detailed what his phobia was like. He approached the classroom, became sick to his stomach, got a blinding headache, and had to

return home. The desensitizer attempted to encourage G to visualize the experience; he was unable to do so and was discharged.
He saw a nutritionist who treated him with various special foods
and vitamins that helped. This was during the summer; he felt
stronger and thought the problem was solved. School began, and
his phobia was even more intense. He saw a third therapist who
directed him to exercise his will power; he felt totally misunder-
stood and left. He was convinced that he had a serious physical
illness, saw his internist, and when G was unable to take a series
of GI tests, the internist made the referral. G then asked the therapist if he could help and if it could be within a few weeks. He
had to take the college test, and there was very little time. The
therapist had been listening and thinking that an extended period
of therapeutic contact would be necessary to effect a change. In
addition, the therapist was considering the separation anxieties
that were inherent in finishing school. The therapist commented
on G's desperation and wondered if he might be asking whether
the therapist would be in a hurry. G's response was to talk about
the exam and its meaning to him. He assumed the therapist
thought he was doing all of this for someone else. The therapist
must think that he was being pressured and that he did not want
to take the exam and did not want to go to college. G wanted to
assure the therapist, with all of his heart and soul, that he wanted
to take the test and go to school. He wanted to be sure that the
therapist understood this. He then wondered if the therapist
meant that there might be something going on inside of him that
he knew nothing about and that the therapist was listening for that
and hearing it. The therapist remarked that G seemed to be saying that he could not hear himself very well and needed help with
that. G agreed, and regular sessions were scheduled.

During the early sessions, G turned to look at the therapist
whenever he spoke and was surprised that his mind was often
blank. He always had something to say, and this had never hap-
pened to him before. He thought of lying in his bed at night feeling scared that everything was out of control; now he felt scared
because nothing came to his mind. He felt pressure to talk that
reminded him of the time pressure in his life. After a few weeks,
G spoke of feeling more contained and recalled his thoughts when
lying in bed. They were not so jumbled and chaotic but consisted

of his feeling that he was in danger. It was like hearing footsteps and imagining that something was threatening you that could not be seen. In feeling contained, G could represent the threat and was shifting into the position of an object phobia.

The following session occurred just prior to the date of G's college exam. He entered in a state of agitation. He had found a way to take the exams, but it required a note from the therapist. With the note, he could be given the exam by himself and would not have to enter the classroom. He asked if the therapist would write the note, and the therapist simply remarked, ''Let's see what comes to mind.'' G thought of one example after another of being put down and being considered incapable of any accomplishment. Whenever he completed a task, it was diminished. He launched into an angry tirade against his parents. His father was unappreciative and could never allow any show of feeling. His mother was constantly critical of him and considered him incapable of any achievement. G was constantly criticized by both parents for being weak and infantile. G stopped and asked, ''You haven't answered me; what about the note?'' The therapist stated that G seemed to be asking whether the therapist considered him to be ineffective. G fell silent and expressed a tremendous feeling of disappointment. He had found a way to take the test, and the therapist's words were implying he would not sign the note. The therapist seemed to think that signing the note would be like ensuring that G remain inept. At the end of the session, G looked at the therapist and stated, ''I guess what you are really saying is, I'll have to wait and see what I do about the exam. If I really trust myself, whether I take it or not is not important. It's what I do that's important, and I need to understand that.''

That night the therapist received a call from G's parents. He had just stormed out of the house, and they wanted advice as to what to do. The therapist simply stated he could not talk. This session took place 2 days later. G began by referring to his parents' call and the therapist's response. He had left his session and was typing an essay about what it meant to look at your life in a new way. He was reminded of a book he read and of his identification with one of the characters who had done something beautiful. He had followed his heart. However, it had so offended society that the wrath of society descended upon him and led to his death. He was writing the essay to put into words what it meant to follow his heart. As he typed, his mother asked him to do a chore. He continued to type and she pulled out the sheet. He exploded, pushed her, felt devastated, and ran out of the house to be alone. He was affected by the dawning realization that powerful emotions were present deep within him and that they were creating his symptom. The character in the book touched him so deeply that he could not get it out of his mind. He was aware of his feelings in a way that he had never experienced before and had never been able to put into words. When it was quiet, he could feel the voice of his mother inside of him saying, ''I am going to engulf you; I am going to kill you.'' It made him feel like he would die or kill himself. His nausea felt like he was trying to get rid of these frightening inner sensations but could not. It felt like he was attached to them and to his father and mother in ways that he could not let go of or digest. He began to think of the book and noted that he had not mentioned the details. He wanted to believe the therapist knew the story so he would not have to talk about it. He sensed that the specifics were connected to a vulnerable and sensitive part of himself that was just beginning to develop and grow. It felt so vulnerable that if he talked about it, he would draw back instead of being able to grow. *G* fell silent. He then stated that the character he identified with had a sexual relationship with the wife of a lordly figure, who became pregnant and had a baby. *G* saw the husband much as he saw his father and himself as having some kind of hidden and special relationship with his mother. *G* now mentioned a younger brother for the first time. He watched his brother and mother, and they seemed to have a very special bond that gave *G* an eerie feeling. It felt like he had either wanted such a relationship and embraced it vicariously or that sometime in his life he might have been involved in the same way. He felt scared in thinking about it.

A shift had taken place from a self-phobia to an object phobia, and instinctual representation had continued to a genital consolidation with the elaboration of an oedipal conflict. Previously, the anxiety associated with an oedipal situation had been so overwhelming that the developmental step to object relatedness could not be negotiated. The threat to cohesiveness that it entailed had instigated a regression to a narcissistically determined self-phobic structural organization.

The Combined Self- and Object Phobias

The following example is of a child primarily exhibiting the structural organization of a combined self- and object phobia. The fixation points on both the projective and introjective arms of perception are threatened with dissolution; there is a phobic attitude toward the influences of a bad object and toward instinctual over-stimulation; and there is little capacity for symbolic representation. The phobia is experienced as a vague inner sense of dread usually linked to an environmental stimulus. The dependency upon external objects for regulation is at its height, and there is a potential for momentary episodes of loss of cohesiveness.

H was an 11-year-old girl referred from another city. The family was moving and wanted assurance that their child would have a therapist. The father called to ask if the child could meet the therapist before they moved, and the therapist agreed. The night before, a message was left canceling the appointment. Several months later, the father called to make an appointment for the mother, father, and child to meet with the therapist. *H* spoke to the therapist on the phone and said it was her idea to have her parents come in because she was scared about meeting the therapist. She could only come in if they came with her. She added that she had insisted on coming several months ago but at the last minute decided not to. An appointment was made, and all three arrived.

H was an uncoordinated, gangly girl who looked out of place. Her parents were well dressed, intellectual, and sophisticated. *H* looked disheveled, sloppy, and awkward. She appeared shy and frightened. The parents began by complaining about coming. *H* had been in therapy before; the family had moved, which was traumatic for her, and they had tried to soften the blow by telling *H* they would find someone for her. *H* was smiling shyly. The therapist asked if *H* felt able to talk alone. She immediately ordered her parents to "go away." She spoke immediately of her previous therapist. He was marvelous, and she missed him. It was hard to leave him because he was so understanding. She did not think she could tolerate the separation, but now she felt OK about it. The therapist seemed friendly and she liked the sound of his voice. She could just tell the therapist would be a nice person, and she felt tremendously relieved. She went on to talk of how uprooted she felt—from friends, school, and neighborhood. *H* spoke in detail of her neighborhood. She knew every corner of it. It was all open to her, and she always knew where she could find her parents. She knew everyone, and everyone knew her parents. She was fearful of being in strange territory. *H* then asked if the therapist knew her previous therapist and went on to describe the good things he did. His office was in a shopping area; her parents left her and went shopping, and she did not feel left out because he bought her treats. *H* hoped the therapist would do likewise and was suddenly concerned that she could not remember what her previous therapist looked like. It scared her.

Consciously, *H* was demanding to be fed, stimulated, regulated, and comforted. This seemed to be her way of gaining regulation and of easing the anxiety of separation. Yet she could not retain the image of the therapist who participated in this manner. *H* appeared to display the fixed phobic attitude toward instinctual overstimulation and toward the influences of a bad object that are characteristic of a combined self- and object phobia.

The therapist commented that he thought *H* was concerned that he would do these things and prevent her from feeling. *H*'s immediate reaction was to state, ''Do you mean you will not get me gifts or presents?''; she then proceeded to talk about her life being dominated by housekeepers and cooks. They were always coming and going. She constantly experienced separations from people who were responsible for her care. A new one arrived, she formed an attachment, and then they left. At the end of the session, the therapist introduced the question of scheduling regular times, and *H* wanted to meet every day. However, she went on to describe situations in which she was appeased and infantilized. This reminded her of how hard she worked and of the little time she had for herself. The therapist stated he thought this was a message that *H* needed some time by herself, and he arranged sessions on alternate days.

During the ensuing months, several themes emerged. *H* talked much about how overworked she was and of the inordinate demands that were constantly placed upon her. People expected far too much. The therapist, in hearing this theme, thought of it as a derivative expressing *H*'s response to his attitude. Any comment that these expressions had reference to *H*'s feeling about the therapist would elicit an immediate response of denial, "Oh no, it's not about you." *H* would go on to emphasize how she only had the most positive of feelings toward the therapist. She saw the therapist as being the most understanding, kind, and warm person. Another theme was of being a scapegoat, particularly in her family, but also in school. If anyone had a bad day, it was blamed upon her. She described parental fights and her efforts to stop them. These eventuated in her being attacked and blamed for the disturbance. She was constantly seen as the source of all troubles, regardless of their nature. Another theme was of leaving her old neighborhood. This was associated with an intense and tearful feeling of longing. Her descriptions were elaborate and created an image of a communal environment that offered containment, pleasure, and a joyful sharing of experience with the parental presence always available. She was tearful as she talked about the loss and had the feeling it could never be regained.

H's longing for the old neighborhood and the extreme disruption created by the move seemed to reflect a traumatic period of her early development. There was a dramatic change in the maternal attitude toward her with the birth of a sibling at age 10 months. It was reminiscent of a feature frequently present as a contributing factor in phobic pathology. There is a well-contained, empathic environment in the early oral phase that is suddenly disrupted as individuation is beginning to arise. The change instigates a premature search for the impressions of a good object, and differentiation is maintained by a phobic attitude toward the representation of an orally determined bad incorporative object.

A new theme then emerged, which concerned people who left her upon short notice. She stressed that the traumatic aspect was not the separation itself but the lack of notice so as to have time to prepare and react. The therapist discovered, just prior to the following session, that he would be out of town and miss a session with *H* at the end of the week.

H began by talking about her outrage at people who left without notice. She spoke of her father who suddenly stated he would be away. Her mother often left and did not let her know until the night before. A housekeeper was leaving and only informed her at the last minute. A teacher was pregnant and let her know one day before departing. The therapist stated that *H* was talking of her feeling about people's leaving without notice and that something had come up that made it necessary for the therapist to miss a session. *H* looked surprised and began to say that was OK, and she mumbled that she knew the therapist could not help it. She paused and asked, "Will you make up the time?" She went on to indicate all of the ways in which the time could be made up and rescheduled. The therapist stated that he did not want to answer until he and *H* had a clearer picture of what that would mean to her. She said it was essential to have the time made up and remembered numerous examples of her parents buying her presents whenever they left that made up for the leaving. She felt better about it, was not so upset, and even looked forward to the present when they were away. *H* stopped and stated, "Oh, I know you won't get me a present. That isn't what I want. I just want you to make up the time." She emphasized its importance in preventing her from getting angry and upset. The session was ending, and she asked, "Well, will you make up the time?" The therapist remarked that he would not make up the time. *H* exploded in rage; her face became red, and she pulled at her hair. She stormed out, slamming the door, and shouted, "I hate you!"

In an object phobia, there is enough stability for the threat to cohesiveness by the influences of a bad object to be symbolically represented and for instinctual activity to expand toward a genital consolidation. The fixation point on the projective arm of perception is in danger of losing its stabilizing function, and psychic activity is inhibited within the system of object representations. The phobic attitude is in response to stimuli evocative of a bad object's influence. When the increase in instinctual activity reaches traumatic proportions, there is a shift to a self-phobic structural organization. The fixation point on the introjective arm of perception is threatened with dissolution, and psychic activity is limited within the self-system of representations. The stress at the fixation point on the projective arm of perception is temporarily alleviated, which enables psychic content to be elaborated in the object system. The phobic attitude is in response to instinctual overstimulation. In the combined self- and object phobias, cohesiveness is threatened by the influences of a bad object and by instinctual overstimulation, and there is little capacity for elaborating psychic content in either system. The phobic attitude is in response to all stimuli possessing bad qualities, which must then be avoided. Pressure is exerted upon external objects to reinforce this narcissistically fixated defensive position. Kohut (1971) referred to this phenomena as an expression of narcissistic transferences that had to be encouraged to further developmental progression. The therapist can then be utilized as a self-object for mirroring or idealization in order to heal defects in the self. This conception places too great an emphasis upon conscious empathy and tends to obscure the guidance available to a therapist from the activity of unconscious perceptions. In addition, idealizations are an attempt to compensate for deficiencies by attributing qualities that are needed to an object. *H*'s idealizations of the therapist expressed the nature of her deficiencies. She consistently portrayed the therapist as kind, understanding, and well contained, specifically idealizing qualities that involved an absence of aggression. She phobically avoided any self-experiences of aggression and of experiencing an object as incorporative or impinging. Objects were almost exclusively portrayed as abandoning and unempathic. The therapist intervened by refusing to participate in reinforcing *H*'s narcissistically fixated pathological defense, and her response was to become enraged. Although *H* was filled with aggression, she did not perceive the therapist as a phobic object, indicating some available capacity for instinctual representation.

H came to her next session looking very excited, which was quite unusual for her. She could not wait to tell the therapist what had occurred the previous evening. She began by referring to her fear of being in the house alone. At those times, she was filled with a vague, ill-defined, ominous sense of dread in response to the stimuli of her environment–thunder, storms, darkness, wind, noises in the house, and the like. Everyone had left the house; she was thinking about her session and about how furious she was. She had never felt that way before and began to worry that the therapist would not see her or that she would be too humiliated to come back. She remembered getting angry, and it felt like she would burst. At that moment, there was a burst of light. It seemed to be outside of her, like the lights of a passing car. She felt like she was about to be attacked and was terrified. Suddenly, she knew it was her grandmother's spirit. Her grandmother had died when *H* was 10 months old and was especially important to her. She died at the time of her sister's birth; she had never known her sister, which made *H* special to the grandmother. At first *H* was terrified, but, as the idea formed that it was her grandmother, the terror subsided. *H* and the grandmother engaged in a dialogue inside of *H*. The grandmother wanted to know about her life and what she was doing. *H* told the grandmother of her complaints, of being scapegoated, and of people leaving her. The grandmother stated that she had to develop her own life and that she could not be so dependent. The grandmother told *H* to let go of her hold on others so that she did not have to depend on their behavior for her well-being. The grandmother was portrayed as a pragmatic, understanding figure who placed emphasis on autonomy and independence. *H* was excited at having this image inside of her, which felt like a helpful presence.

H had established cohesiveness on the basis of a phobic attitude toward the influences of a bad object and toward instinctual overstimulation. She was confronted with the constant pressure of an overloading of aggression, and her entire attitude was focused upon preventing any awareness of its magnitude. The therapist's refusal to participate in reinforcing her defensive posture enabled the underlying aggression to be expressed and represented. The object impressions of the therapeutic interaction were now available as a source of restraint and regulation; this was reflected in the representation of the grandmother. This figure embodied the qualities she had experienced in the relationship with the therapist and facilitated a rapid shift to the structural organization of an object phobia. *H* was displaying the capacity to symbolically represent the threat to cohesiveness by the influences of a bad object, with the momentary terror at the sense of being overwhelmed. She was also giving evidence of a beginning superego consolidation as the terror subsided and as a helpful regulating presence took its place. The phobic attitude that had dominated her life was alleviated, and it was now possible for advances in instinctual representation to be effected.

Summary

A point is reached within the narcissistically organized personality when no additional instinctual representation can take place. At this juncture, instinctual demand of any greater intensity poses a threat to cohesiveness, and a phobic situation is created. Further progression can not transpire until new structures develop. It is this phobic situation that motivates a shift from narcissism to object relatedness, organized around the fulcrum of an oedipal conflict. The phobias are disorders in which that shift has begun to occur and in which the individual has been overwhelmed by the increase in instinctual activity associated with the oedipal situation. The response is to defensively regress to a narcissistic fixation. The particular phobic symptomatology that is manifested fluctuates, depending upon the adaptational demands of the external world and the level of instinctual intensity in the internal world.

The superego organization of the phobic individual is affected by an inability to utilize the process of identification with an aggressor. The orally determined influences of a bad impinging object are devouring rather than restraining and cannot be included within self-experience. The prohibitive function of the superego is ineffective, and the dependency upon external objects for regulation is continued. It is only when the phobic situation is alleviated that the nature of an object's influence can change and identification with an aggressor can become a functional process.

A fantasy that is associated with anxiety does not constitute a phobia. Many fantasies are representative of instinctual conflict, are associated with anxiety, and have been labeled as *phobias*. Phobias are indicative of a limited ability to represent instinctual demand; the anxiety is of panic proportions; and they are characterized by avoidance. There are many individuals, with fantasies associated with anxiety, that have a hysteric or obsessive structural foundation. The particular fantasies (a fear of flying, or of the water, etc.) do not necessitate an avoidance of the stimuli that evoke them. The concept of a counterphobic defense is often utilized to explain how such individuals can place themselves in a phobic situation. Counterphobic maneuvers are certainly observable in a large number of patients. This phenomenon is an adaptive response to an external situation that is evocative of an anxiety-laden fantasy. The individual, either in defense by denial, or to attain mastery, deliberately confronts an anxiety-arousing situation. Body ego experiences result that amplify the representation of autonomous ego functions and the background object of primary identification. Perceptual attention is then focused upon these good self-experiences, and the anxiety recedes.

I have utilized examples from pubescent and adolescent patients because the phobic nature of this narcissistic personality disorder is more noticeable and the effects of the therapeutic interaction are more clearly demonstrable over a shorter span of time. Unconsciously, empathic communications are evocative of the impressions of a good object, which provides the stability that facilitates representation of instinctual activity. In these phobic disorders, the increase in instinctual activity associated with the oedipal situation has been overwhelming and has instigated a narcissistically fixated regression. Instinctual expansion can only be manifested when the influences of a good object are amplified to stabilize cohesiveness and alleviate a phobic situation.

Phobic individuals possess an exquisite reactive sensitivity to the qualities of an interaction. The manner in which cohesiveness is structured has left little capacity for extensive representational activity in the self- and object systems. When the stimuli of an interaction are not unconsciously empathic, they are immediately evocative of the phobically avoided influences of a bad object. The object in the external world is then perceived as a potentially threatening figure that must be avoided. This response is a transference distortion but is instigated by an unconscious perception. Individuals with this structural makeup can only adapt to an impinging stimulus by avoidance. Lapses in empathy are an inevitable occurrence in any therapeutic interaction. However, if the phobic response is understood as a distortion rather than the consequence of an unconscious perception, the developmental trauma is perpetuated, and the phobic situation is intensified. When a phobic response is recognized as evidence of an unconscious perception of unempathic qualities in the interaction, the source can be identified. Individuals with a greater capacity for representation can respond to lapses in empathy in a variety of ways, but the phobic individual can only respond by avoidance. *F*, for example, stated that he had to have a good reason. That is, an external object had to bring something (a reason) that evoked an inner experience that was not previously present (an increase in representation). He could listen to "good reasons" because they were responsive to internal experiences that he had not been aware of before. The phobic individual is limited in the capacity to represent derivatives, and a phobic response can serve as a guide. In all three examples when the therapist was unconsciously empathic, cohesiveness was stabilized, the phobic situation was alleviated, a fuller capacity to represent instinctual activity emerged, and intrapsychic conflict became more evident.

The Structure of Thought in the Phobic Disorders

The following thought, expressed in a clinical situation, will be examined to determine the underlying structural organization of the personality. It includes a reference to the conditions that were present prior to a therapeutic relationship and gives some indication of its effects.

"I want to go back to where we left off. It reminds me of falling asleep. Falling asleep and not being able to get out. A long time ago, I talked about how much trouble I had falling asleep."

The statement begins with: "I want to go back to where we left off." This embodies a representation of the self clearly united with and differentiated from an object. It depicts the self as having been away from the object and expresses a wish to return to a previous and different relationship. The portrayal of a well-differentiated self and object and of a connection between them reflects the presence of cohesiveness.

Developmentally, once cohesiveness has been established, there are two situations that can encompass this quality of engagement with an object. One involves the self's reacting to the impingements of an object and moving away. However, the thought gives no indication of an impingement, and the wish to return to the object implies an absence of impinging qualities. The second set of conditions, in which the self is represented as leaving the object, involves the process of forming a fixation point on the introjective arm of perception. The structuralization of the ego ideal, based upon selective identifications, has directed the focus of perceptual attention upon the representations of self-experience. The subsequent recognition of the good self's bad instinctual qualities establishes a fixation point on the introjective arm of perception. Perceptual attention has shifted from the impressions of an object to self-experience, which is consistent with the idea of having been with the object and left. We can speculate that the wish to return to a previous position was the result of recognizing a potentially traumatic instinctual self-experience.

The return to a previous level of organization involves a regressive movement, which is mediated by the functions of the grandiose self and ego ideal. When these unifying and differentiating structures are composed of differing facets of an object's influence, regressive movements meet with oppositional forces. The ease and readiness with which this regressive return is considered would require the grandiose self and ego ideal to be interrelated in their functioning, as is characteristic of the phobic disorders. The capacity to negotiate a progressive movement away from the object to recognize the good self's bad instinctual qualities and to regress to a previous position necessitates that the structures of the grandiose self and ego ideal be a unified functional entity. The statement continues, "It reminds me of falling asleep." The focused perceptual functions of the eye of consciousness are suspended in the process of falling asleep, and the perceptual functions of the superego eye assume dominance. These are the perceptual functions incorporated in the structuralization of the grandiose self and ego ideal. The statement, "It reminds me of falling asleep," appears to reflect a reactive sensitivity to the similarity in the process of falling asleep and the position that is sought with the object.

The remainder of the thought gives an indication of the nature of the original pathology and of the effects of the therapeutic relationship. It refers to a previous difficulty in falling asleep and to a change after therapy was initiated. The original, more extreme pathology is hinted at by the following statement: "Falling asleep and not being able to get out." This represents the self's being trapped inside of an object, which reflects the impression of an orally incorporative, bad impinging object. The change is implied in the ability to fall alseep and to leave the object. The hypothesis is that prior to psychotherapy, the developmental step of forming a fixation point on the introjective arm of perception was only accomplished with an inordinate degree of trauma. In that previous structural position, it was frightening to fall asleep. The fixation points on both arms of perception were highly unstable, and the predominant structural organization appeared to be that of a combined self- and object phobia. The perceptual functions of the eye of consciousness could not be completely suspended in the process of falling asleep. With therapy, falling asleep is no longer traumatic. In addition, there is an advance toward recognizing the good self's bad instinctual qualities, although with difficulty. The continuing presence of phobic pathology is indicated by the characteristic relationship of the grandiose self and the ego ideal, but we can postulate that progression toward object relatedness has become possible. The therapeutic relationship appears to have amplified and expanded the impressions of a good object's influence, which have increased their availability for the process of selective identification. The ego ideal has then become more effective in strengthening the stability of self-experience.

In health, developmental progression is anxiety relieving because a greater degree of stability is attained. Regression involves a loss of function, which is anxiety arousing. In pathology, developmental progression is anxiety arousing because stability is threatened. Regression is associated with a reduction of anxiety. The exception involves those pathological constellations wherein a regression is out of control, rather than being in the service of defense. The statement reflects an increase in anxiety with progression and a reduction in anxiety with regression, indicative of the defensive significance of the regression.

CHAPTER 11

The Cohesive Disorders
A Comparison

This chapter will summarize and compare the pathological entities that occur within a cohesively organized personality. The comparison focuses attention upon those areas of psychological
functioning that have particular relevance for a therapeutic relationship. All mental activity is determined by the representations
of self-experience and of an object's influence that are at its foundation. The significance of the developmental events that have
shaped the formation of pathological distortions is an essential in-
gredient for broadening the capacity for a therapeutic response and
for gaining a fuller awareness of the effects of a therapeutic en-
counter. Psychological functioning encompasses an intermingling
of healthy and pathological forces, and the comparison will include
the healthy outcome of the genital character as a background.

The Self-Representational System

The self-representational system includes the body ego experiences of instinctual activity, the exercise of autonomous functions, the background object of primary identification, sensory
deprivations, and reactions to impingement. It is the source of in-
itiative, contains the representations of fusion and merger that are
structured to absorb narcissistic injuries or exert a regressive pull,
is utilized in the formation of conversion symptoms, and is a foundation for processes of introjection. Entities of good self-experience

not requiring defense and of bad self-experience requiring defense are connected by a line of continuity in the realm of instinctual experience.

The Genital Character

There is a balanced progression in the representation of libidinal activity through the advancing phases of psychosexual development. Sublimated expressions of the component instincts are manifested under the special conditions of play, regression in the service of the ego, and empathic experiences. The consolidation of the component instincts into a genital drive culminates in the formation and resolution of an oedipal conflict, which creates a structured pathway of instinctual integration. A continuous influx of instinctual demand has access to processes of sublimation and secondary autonomy; this adds vitality to all experience. A genitally determined, object-related orientation predominates and enhances the continuing expansion of the personality. A new object-related boundary for the system of unconscious mental activity is well established, and its function is silently present. Aggression is differentiating in its effects, and well-balanced proportions of sensory deprivations and reactions to impingement are available for defensive purposes.

The Hysterias

Hysterical disorders have a characteristic configuration in the self-representational system. Instinctual experiences are unbalanced, with an emphasis on the oral and phallic aspects. The autonomous ego functions are diminished, the background object of primary identification firm and stable, sensory deprivations are excessive, and the reactions to impingement are hypertrophied. Sensory deprivations and reactions to impingement are involved in the formation of defensive structures, which are designed to regulate the phallic and genital overstimulations that are consistently present.

The genital fantasy elaborations of the oedipal conflict may attain some degree of partial resolution, which is accompanied by the formation of symptomatic compromises. These hysterical conversion symptoms, which give expression to defensively disguised instinctual activity, are founded upon the representations of self-experience. The structured pathway of instinctual integration is intermittently functional, operates as a stimulus for defensive opposition, and does not allow a continuous, uninterrupted flow of instinctual demand. The genitally determined structure forming the boundary of the unconscious system of mental activity is periodically active, as the need for defensive regulation is intensified. When hysterical character pathology predominates, the effects of a fixed, phallically determined influence upon perception create some differences. Identifications with a phallically humiliating aggressor are more active, and the reaction formations they establish within self-experience act as a powerful prohibitive force. The structured pathway of instinctual integration is more heavily defended against, the oedipal conflict remains unresolved, and the boundary of the unconscious system (manifested by incestuous fantasies) is overdeveloped.

The Obsessives

Obsessive forms of pathologies are characterized by their emphasis upon anality. Anal instinctual experiences are enormously overdeveloped and exert an ongoing influence upon phallic and genital instinctual expansion. Good qualities of mastery and control are stressed, whereas bad qualities are vigorously defended against. These bad qualities are represented as sadistic, reflecting the overloading of aggression and inadequate fusion of libidinal and aggressive drives. The autonomous ego functions are over-extended, the background object of primary identification is firm, and sensory deprivations and reactions to impingement are diminished.

The fixation point on the introjective arm of perception, based upon the recognition of the good self's bad anal instinctual qualities, remains unintegrated. It is at the foundation of the fixed character attitudes designed to maintain internal regulation. Obsessive character pathology is dominated by thc effects of reaction formations, which are created by identification with an anally sadistic aggressor. The experiences of disgust, shame, and guilt are mobilized in response to instinctual activity, to guard against the emergence of anal sadism. The structured pathway of instinctual integration is heavily defended, and the boundary of the unconscious system is consistently active. These object-related structures, formed by the organizing function of the oedipal conflict, have a strong anal-genital composition.

The intensity of anally influenced instinctual demands may lead to a regressive breakdown in function of the fixation point on the introjective arm of perception. Obsessive symptoms are then formed in an attempt to achieve regulation. These are compromises involving the expression of instinctual demand in defensively disguised form and include a superego response. They exist on a hierarchy from intrusive ideation through behavioral rituals to compulsive acts. To the extent that ideational components predominate, the symptoms are primarily manifested within the object system of representations. When body ego experiences are involved in the symptomatic compromise, as is the case with tics and hand-washing compulsions, it is an indication of an inordinate degree of stress. In the presence of symptoms, the structures that form a pathway of instinctual integration are heavily defended, intermittently disruptive, and instigate the formation of new symptoms.

The Phobias

The phobias are narcissitically determined and object-related disorders, and they exhibit shifts and fluctuations from one phobic attitude to another. An object phobia, self-phobia, or combined self- and object phobia may be manifested, depending upon whether it is the influence of an object or instinctual overstimulation that is threatening cohesiveness. In all, there is a pattern of instinctual imbalance that is a product of trauma at the point of individuation. The early oral dimensions of good instinctual self-experience are abundant and abruptly diminish, whereas bad instinctual experience is minimal in its early oral aspects and extensively represented during the later period of orality. This oral aggressive influence is exerted upon any anal, phallic, or genital expansion that transpires. Autonomous ego functions are hypertrophied, and the background object of primary identification is fairly stable. Sensory deprivations and reactions to impingement are uneven, being minimally represented in the early oral period and vastly expanded in the ensuing phases of development.

In the object phobias, instinctual experience may expand to encompass anal and phallic sensations and even extend to the beginnings of a genital consolidation. Those aspects not requiring defense are minimal, overstimulation is a constant threat, and the influence of oral aggression is extreme. The symbolic representation of the particular object phobia offers some degree of regulation, but any emerging oedipal constellation jeopardizes the stabilizing function of the fixation point on the introjective arm of perception. The boundary of the unconscious system continues to be maintained by the narcissistically determined structure of impingements and the reactions to them. The self-phobias embody the same pattern of representation in the self-system; the only difference is in the limitations in expansion of instinctual representation and the absence of the object phobia. In the combined self- and object phobias, instinctual representation remains at the level of orality, and the background object of primary identification may exhibit some instability. There is also evidence of stress on the lines of cleavage delineating the varying aspects of self-experience; this is expressed in the anxiety of fragmentation.

The Object Representational System

The object representational system includes the object-impression counterparts of self-experience that are utilized in structuralizing cohesiveness, in compensatory mechanisms, in strengthening differentiation and self-regulation, and in establishing a foundation for projective processes. Entities of a good object's influence and a bad object's influence are connected by a line of continuity in the realm of prohibitive experience.

The Genital Character

The representations of an object, both good and bad, are well modulated and reflect a balanced progression through the advancing phases of psychosexual development. The impressions of a good, anally derived instinctual object are elaborated into fantasies of omnipotence, which are embodied in the structure of the grandiose self. The ego ideal has been primarily structured by including the influences of a phallically determined, optimally frustrating good object within self-experience. The infantile representations of an object, upon which these differentiating structures have been based, have been replaced by the impressions of new and independent objects. The grandiose self and ego ideal then operate as boundaries, within which the superego is consolidated as an independently functioning agency. The genital, instinctual impressions of a bad object are elaborated into primal scene fantasies, which are structurally united with the representations of bad instinctual self-experience to form a pathway of integration. This structure functions in a fluid and continuous fashion, with only minimal defensive opposition. The process of identification with an aggressor is functional under stress, and aggression provides a differentiating, regulatory influence rather than a destructive one. The process of depersonification is ongoing and effective, and the mechanisms of projection involved in language, symbol formation, conceptualization, and internal thought are functional and expansive.

The Hysterias

The representation of a good object is imbalanced, with the oral and phallic instintual aspects disproportionately expanded and the optimally frustrating aspects relatively sparse. The impressions of a good phallic instinctual object are elaborated into fantasies of an admiring audience and structuralize the grandiose self. The optimally frustrating influences of an object are too deficient and do not provide sufficient restraint to be major components of the ego ideal. The phallically humiliating impressions of an impinging bad object are predominantly selected to form that differentiating structure. The grandiose self and ego ideal retain their infantile attachments, and the superego is not fully integrated with the interests of the ego. The representation of a bad object is also imbalanced, with the oral and phallic instinctual aspects excessive and the depriving and impinging aspects overemphasized. Genital primal scene fantasies, reflecting the functioning of a structured pathway of integration, are intermittently active and defensively opposed.

Incestuous fantasies, reflecting the defensive functions of the boundary of the unconscious system, are intermittently active and quiescent. When hysterical character pathology is in evidence, incestuous fantasies predominate to the exclusion of primal scene fantasies.

The Obsessives

The optimally gratifying instinctual representation of a good object is diminished in its oral aspects, excessive in its anal qualities, and anally influenced in its phallic and genital dimensions. Optimally frustrating impressions are hypertrophied. The impressions of a good, anally derived instinctual object are elaborated into fantasies of omnipotence, which structuralize the grandiose self. This is similar to what takes place in healthy development, although the anal qualities are more archaic and the omnipotence more extreme. The ego ideal has been primarily structured by including the sadistically impinging influences of a bad object within self-experience, due to the inordinate need for harsh prohibitions. The grandiose self and ego ideal retain their infantile attachments, and the superego remains harshly punitive at an immature level of organization. The representation of a bad object displays the overriding impact of anality, with the instinctual aspect's giving emphasis to anal subjugation and control and the impinging aspect's being anally sadistic. The impressions of a depriving object are relatively diminished and are represented as anally withholding. Anally influenced, genital primal scene fantasies are actively defended against, and anal-genital incestuous fantasies predominate.

When there has been a regressive breakdown in the effectiveness of anally determined character fixations, obsessive symptoms are formed. Representations of an object are included in the symptomatic compromises, and compensatory idealizations are more in evidence. Anal-genital primal scene fantasies, which are so vigorously defended against when character pathology is manifested, become periodically active and disruptive. They operate to instigate an escalation in the formation of symptoms. The instrusive quality of obsessive symptoms is a reflection of the breakdown in defense.

The Phobias

The representation of a good optimally gratifying instinctual object is hypertrophied in its early oral qualities and then abruptly diminished. This early oral influence is overvalued and powerful, affecting all further expansion into anal, phallic, and genital impressions of optimal gratification. Early impressions of an optimally frustrating object are adequately represented but cannot be enlarged because of their evocative connection to early trauma and to the phobically avoided impressions of an orally incorporative bad object. The impressions of a good orally derived instinctual object are elaborated into fantasies of an all-giving nurturer, which structuralize the grandiose self. The ego ideal is structured by including the influences of an optimally gratifying, orally determined object within self-experience. The grandiose self and ego ideal, in being composed of the same aspect of an object's influence, are contiguous in their functioning and highly unstable. The superego is ineffective in its prohibitive and guiding functions, and the dependency upon external objects for regulation is exaggerated. The representation of a bad object has a dominant oral influence, with early oral qualities diminished and a sudden hypertrophy during the later oral period. The impinging impression of a bad object is orally incorporative in nature and exerts a threat to maintaining cohesiveness at the fixation point on the projective arm of perception. The capacity for object-related perceptions has not been structured, and the boundary of the unconscious system is maintained by impingements and the reactions to them. In the self-phobias, the threat to cohesiveness by instinctual overstimulation is symbolically represented as being trapped and immobilized in an enclosed space that must be avoided.

Self–Object Need

Self–object need refers to the particular qualities needed from an external object to either further developmental progression or to reinforce pathological defenses.

The Genital Character

Self–object needs are numerous and varied. They center upon the self-enhancement that results from the ability to love an object and are manifested in an increasing engagement with object-related attachments.

The Hysterias

The presence of hysterical symptoms is indicative of a greater degree of advancement toward object relatedness, and the self–object need is for optimally frustrating qualities in an interaction to further the thrust of developmental progression. It is this quality that has been relatively deficient and is a factor in the unrealized potentials that are an integral part of this disorder.

When hysterical character pathology is manifested, the self–object need is expressed in the pressure exerted upon external objects to reinforce fixed phallically determined attitudes. This takes the form of recreating an interaction that elicits a humiliating aggressive response to the expression of phallic exhibitionism. This is often referred to as the ''seductiveness'' of the hysteric.

The Obsessives

The self–object need in obsessive character pathology is for reinforcement of fixed anally determined attitudes. This takes the form of recreating sadomasochistic qualities in an interaction. When a regressive breakdown results in the formation of obsessive symptoms, an effort is made to gain control over all external objects.

The Phobias

The object phobias have a self–object need for idealizations, which offer some degree of stability to the tenuously maintained fixation point on the projective arm of perception. The self-phobias seek out interactions that regulate instinctual activity and that are restrictive or inhibitory. In the combined self- and object phobias, the self–object need is for optimally gratifying, optimally frustrating, orally nurturing interactions. There is also a high investment in maintaining prolonged contact with transitional objects.

The Nature of Anxiety and Repression

The Genital Character

There are transient episodes of anxiety in response to superego disapproval. The structure of castration anxiety is functional, serves as a source of internal regulation, and operates to signal for the institution of defensive responses and integrative processes. Repression proper is well established, is invoked at the source of stimulation, and the superego is integrated and harmoniously functional with the interests of the ego.

The Hysterias

The primary anxiety is of castration. The structure of castration anxiety is actively invoked in response to instinctual overstimulation, and it is effective in its signaling function. Repression proper is well established, but perceptual attention continues to be directed away from the source of a threatening stimulus. The ultimate source of overstimulation is the instinctual aspect of a bad object. In hysteria, the object system of representations is underdeveloped, and the effects of an overstimulating bad object resonate throughout, whereas the system of self-representations is overemphasized, and defensive responses are readily accessible. Perceptual attention is thus focused upon the self-system. When hysterical symptoms are in evidence, there has been some limited degree of oedipal conflict resolution and some integration of superego functions. There may be intermittent periods of registering new object-related experiences, supported by the regulatory effect of hysterical symptoms in managing the potential state of overstimulation. This does not occur with hysterical character pathology, in which the superego functions remain polarized and act in opposition to the interests of the ego.

The Obsessives

The primary anxiety is a loss of the love of the object, which reflects the effects of an overloading of aggression. Castration anxiety is functional as a signaling and regulatory structure and is dominated by anally influenced prohibitive responses. Reaction formations, based on identifications with an anal-sadistic aggressor, are a predominant feature and indicative of the immature level of superego organization. In the obsessive, the object system of representations is overdeveloped, and defensive responses are readily accessible, whereas the system of self-representations is poorly regulated and resonates with the impact of an overstimulating instinctual object. The primary source of danger is within the realm of instinctual self-experience, and repression proper functions to direct perceptual attention to the object system. Obsessive symptoms represent an attempt to regulate instinctual activity when there has been a regressive breakdown in the effectiveness of repression proper.

The Phobias

The primary anxiety is of loss of the object, which reflects the instability of the structures maintaining cohesiveness. Repression proper is in the earliest stages of emerging as the primary defensive activity of the ego. In the object phobias, castration anxiety has only tenuously formed and has not solidified as a structure capable of a signaling function. The superego is inadequately consolidated, remaining primarily in the form of its precursors. The influences of a bad, orally incorporative object pose a threat to cohesiveness and are phobically avoided. In the self-phobias, castration anxiety is unformed, and the superego is present only in the form of its precursors. The threat to cohesiveness has shifted, and instinctual overstimulation must be phobically avoided. In the combined self- and object phobias, there is a threat to cohesiveness at both the introjective and projective arms of perception; this necessitates a phobic avoidance of the influences of a bad object and instinctual overstimulation.

The Conflict-Free Sphere

The Genital Character

The final step of a structured pathway of instinctual integration has been negotiated, and the unseen dimensions of instinctual demand have attained secondary autonomy. They are available to form an inner boundary for a conflict free sphere of ego functions. The representations of empathic, object-related contact with separate, independent objects is available to form its outer boundary. There is a well-formed system of conflict-free functions with structured boundaries that facilitate more effective conscious control over the selection of new experiences. The interests of the ego are harmonious with a fully integrated superego.

The Hysterias

The regulatory function of symptoms enables a conflict-free sphere to be intermittently functional with some element of harmony with the superego. However, it is unreliable and easily disrupted by the readiness with which instinctual activity becomes overstimulating. When hysterical character pathology is manifested, conflict-free functions are sporadic and not organized into a system.

The Obsessives

The inability to negotiate the final step in a structured pathway of instinctual integration has not enabled the formation of boundaries for a conflict-free system of functions. There are periodic experiences of conflict-free functioning but with no organization and no integration with the functions of the superego. When obsessive symptoms are formed, the autonomous ego functions are all enmeshed in conflict.

The Phobias

All autonomous ego functions are occupied in the service of defense and in maintaining cohesiveness.

Transference

Transference reactions are divided into three categories of experience, all of which are on a continuum. These include (1) the character defenses or defenses against the transference, (2) the defense transferences, and (3) the transference. Character defenses are based upon the pregenital, narcissistic attachments to an object and to instinctual experience that anchor object constancy and operate as a foundation for fixed character attitudes. They are expressed in the pressure exerted upon an external object to reinforce a pathological defense. Defense transferences are an amalgam of instinctual demands and their characteristic defensive response as they gain access to representation. Unconscious perceptions and transference fantasy distortions are embedded in these amalgams and expressed through the formation of derivatives. The transference refers to those instinctual demands that are relatively unimpeded by defensive opposition.

The Genital Character

Character defenses are discriminatory and responsive to the adaptive demands of a given situation. The introjective arm of perception is open to register new object-related experiences, with little need for defensive distortion. Defense transferences are manifested at transient moments of stress or overstimulation by derivatives of genital incestuous fantasies. These reflect the heightened defensive response associated with the activity of the boundary of the unconscious system. The transference is manifested by derivatives encompassing a full elaboration of genital primal scene fantasies. It is indicative of the unseen dimension of instinctual demand's being included within self-experience and reflects the functional capacity of a structured pathway of instinctual integration.

The Hysterias

Character defenses in the hysteric with symptoms are designed to express phallic exhibitionism, with the intent of engaging a reflective audience. The readiness for phallic overstimulation readily invokes hysterical character pathology, and pressure is exerted to recreate the humiliations that reinforce reaction formations and strengthen fixed phallically determined attitudes. In the male hysteric, defense transferences encompass the castrative threat associated with a genital instinctual attachment to the primary maternal object. The transference is of a positive oedipal constellation. In the female hysteric, the defense transferences are of a negative oedipal configuration. The transference involves the displacement to the male as a genital instinctual love object.

The Obsessives

Character defenses are designed to attain mastery and control. Pressure is exerted to recreate the experience of submission to a sadistic object, which reinforces identifications with a sadistic aggressor. When obsessive symptoms are formed, the adaptive facet of the compromise expresses an anal-sadistic attack upon external objects. It most frequently takes the form of controlling the object's behavior through the symptom. In the male obsessive, defense transferences are of an anally influenced negative genital oedipal conflict. The transference is of a positive anal-genital constellation. In the female obsessive, defense transferences involve a rapid displacement of anal-genital instinctual interest to the male, as a defense against the negative oedipal situation. The transference is of the development step of a negative oedipal situation, leading toward a displacement to the male with less defensive opposition.

The Phobias

In the object phobias, character defenses are designed to idealize an external object. The male defense transferences expresses the onset of an orally influenced genital negative oedipal conflict, which poses a threat to cohesiveness from the effects of instinctual overstimulation. The transference is of an oral incorporative narcissistically determined threat to cohesiveness. The female defense transference express the threat to cohesiveness of any positive oedipal strivings, and the developmental step of a negative oedipal constellation is phobically avoided. In both, the full elaboration of the genital fantasies of an oedipal conflict is a new development.

In the self-phobias, character defenses are designed to attain regulation of instinctual activity. Defense transferences and transferences are threatening to cohesiveness and are phobically avoided. In the combined self- and object phobias, character defenses are designed to regulate self-esteem through gaining consciously empathic, optimally gratifying responses from an external object. Defense transferences and transferences are phobically avoided.

The Conscious and Preconscious Systems

The conscious and preconscious systems refer to the nature of the mental content that is available to the function of self-observation.

The Genital Character

There is a rich uninhibited interplay of immediate perceptions, conceptualizations, depersonified and symbolic mental productions, derivatives of unconscious mental activity, and a ready availability of imagery and fantasy.

The Hysterias

When hysterical symptoms are present, the capacity to register new object-related stimuli is proportional to the degree of integration of the fixation point on the introjective arm of perception. Immediate perceptions may be available and periodically unavailable. There is a predominance of imagery and body sensations; this is the consequence of an overemphasis upon self-experience. A plethora of instinctual derivatives occupy perceptual attention. When hysterical character pathology predominates, there is a diminution of immediate perceptions and an increase in imagery and body sensations. All stimuli have similar qualities, due to the effects of fixed phallically determined attitudes. The fantasy of emptiness, which functions so well to defend against overstimulation, is frequently evoked.

The Obsessives

An inordinate amount of attention is paid to immediate perceptions, which are colored by the influence of fixed anally determined attitudes. Conceptualizations, intellectualization, and processes of projection are hypertrophied. Instinctual derivatives are diminished, as are body sensations and imagery. When obsessive symptoms have developed, they are a constant preoccupation and are associated with an escalation in ideational activity.

The Phobias

There is a tendency to focus attention upon immediate perceptions, with an alertedness to their potential for creating narcissistic injury. Instinctual derivatives are diminished, and the fantasy of emptiness is accentuated. The particular phobic organization in the forefront determines the symbolic representation of the threat to cohesiveness that has to be avoided. These phobic threats are latently present and noticed intermittently.

Drive Development

The Genital Character

The aggressive and libidinal drives are in balanced proportions. Aggression is differentiating, and genital primacy has been well established. Varying levels of neutralized instinctual energies are available to activate the processes of play, empathy, sublimation, and secondary autonomy.

The Hysterias

There is an imbalance in the distribution of the drives, with an overemphasis upon oral and phallic libidinal experiences. Aggression is differentiating, and a genital consolidation has taken place. However, there is only a limited degree of genital instinctual integration.

The Obsessives

The distribution of the drives is uneven and characterized by the extent to which anality is accentuated. Instinctual expansion into phallic experiences and a genital consolidation transpire under the influence of anality, with little capacity for instinctual integration. There is an overloading of aggression, which is poorly neutralized and tends to be disruptive rather than differentiating. With obsessive symptoms, there is the added dimension of less effective regulation of instinctual activity.

The Phobias

The predominance of orality has an influence on any expansion of instinctual activity that occurs. Libidinal and aggressive drives are poorly fused, oral aggression has a destructive effect, and the libidinal representations of fusion and merger are an active force within the personality.

Regression in the Service of the Ego

The Genital Character

Transient regressions in the service of the ego, essential for an empathic understanding of external objects, are readily available. These regressive movements are also available, as needed, for the processes of play and sublimation.

The Hysterias

The formation of conversion symptoms involves a regression in the service of the ego that enables the thrust for progression in development to continue. However, the regression is a product of conflict and displays little flexibility. There may be some limited capacity for regressions in the service of the ego that are manifested in play and to an extent in processes of sublimation. With hysterical character pathology, regressions in the service of the ego are severely limited because the instinctual activity associated with regression quickly becomes overstimulating.

The Obsessives

The fixed anally derived perceptions and attitudes of obsessive character pathology prevent the process of regression in the service of the ego. With the formation of obsessive symptoms, a regression has taken place, but it is the result of a breakdown in function.

The Phobias

Regression operates solely in the service of defense, and in the object and self-phobias is the major defensive response available. In the combined self- and object phobias, regression is threatening and in danger of being out of control.

Reality Testing (The Fixation Points)

The function of reality testing is a product of the manner in which stimuli are registered and the meaning they are given at various levels of consciousness. The composition and stability of the fixation points are major factors in determining the extent to which new experiences are affected by memory. The fixation point on the projective arm of perception, based upon an infantile attachment to an object, must be retained to anchor object constancy and support projective processes. Its influence upon new experience is diminished as it is gradually depersonified and ultimately replaced with the representations of new independent objects. The fixation point on the introjective arm of perception, based upon infantile instinctual experience, must be integrated and relinquished for new experiences that are free of distortion to be registered.

The Genital Character

The fixation point on the projective arm of perception has expanded, undergone a process of depersonification, and gained independence from the influence of the original infantile narcissistic attachment to an object. The fixation point on the introjective arm of perception has been integrated, is no longer required to maintain stability, and its function has been taken over by the conflict-free sphere. New object-related experiences are enhancing, can be registered without distortion, and are acted upon at all levels of consciousnes to give them richness and depth. Reality testing is effective.

The Hysterias

The fixation point on the projective arm of perception is maintained by a phallically determined infantile attachment to an object possessing bad humiliating qualities, and the process of depersonification is diminished. With hysterical symptoms, the fixation point on the introjective arm of perception is partially integrated and only periodically open to new experiences. At these moments, the potential for overstimulation is at its height, and the phallically determined fixation point on the introjective arm of perception asserts its defensive function. Consequently, there are fluctuations from being sensitive to the overstimulating qualities in an interaction, to being totally insensitive to these very same qualities. Reality testing is intermittently effective and narrow in its scope. With hysterical character pathology, the diminution in processes of depersonification is more extreme; this further diminishes the capacity for concept formation and intellectualization. The introjective arm of perception is fixated by the memory traces of phallically determined infantile instinctual experience's exerting a distorting influence upon all new stimuli.

The Obsessives

The fixation point on the projective arm of perception remains under the influence of an anally derived infantile attachment to an object with bad sadistic qualities. Projective processes and intellectual activities are hypertrophied and only minimally depersonified. The fixation point on the introjective arm of perception is defensively maintained by memory traces of anally determined infantile instinctual experience. All new stimuli are affected by the resulting fixed character attitudes. When there is a regressive breakdown in function of the fixation point on the introjective arm of perception, obsessive symptoms are formed, and new stimuli are registered as a potential source of overstimulation.

The Phobias

In the object phobias, the fixation point on the projective arm of perception is threatened with a loss of its differentiating function by the influences of an orally incorporative object. It is maintained by virtue of a phobic avoidance. The fixation point on the introjective arm of perception is more stabilized and based upon orally determined infantile instinctual experience. The relative instability of this fixation point creates an exquisite reactive sensitivity to the qualities of new stimuli because they are immediately evocative of unconscious perceptions. In the self-phobias, the fixation point on the projective arm of perception is also based upon an infantile attachment to an orally derived object with bad incorporative qualities. However, there has been a minimal degree of depersonification alleviating the immediate threat to cohesiveness. Although it remains unstable, there is some support for psychic content to be elaborated in the object system of representations. The fixation point on the introjective arm of perception is vulnerable to a loss of its stabilizing function from the effects of instinctual overstimulation and is maintained by a phobic avoidance. In the combined self- and object phobias, the fixation points on the projective and introjective arms of perception are both tenuous and vulnerable to a loss of function. There is a reactive sensitivity to all stimuli that resonate with the influences of a bad object or with instinctual overstimulation, because they pose a threat to cohesiveness and must be avoided.

The Ego (The Process of Play)

Manifestations of play are a measure of the ego's flexibility and manner of responding to the expression of the component instincts. The capacity to play reflects the functioning of the grandiose self.

The Genital Character

The transient expression of the full range of component instincts is readily available in play and in sublimatory activities. The grandiose self is structured in a stage- and phase-specific fashion during the more modulated anal phase of psychosexual development. It is based upon participation in a fantasy of the object's omnipotence, is a stable structure, and effectively regulates the temporary regression.

The Hysterias

The regulatory function of hysterical symptoms is sufficient for the oral and anal component instincts to be allowed some expression in play. Phallic instinctual activity rapidly becomes overstimulating, and genital experiences are dangerous and actively defended against. With hysterical character pathology, the range of play is narrow and limited by fixed, phallically determined attitudes. The structuralization of the grandiose self has been delayed until the phallic phase and is based upon participation in the fantasied admiration of the object. Qualities of admiration tend to encourage exhibitionism, which is already poorly regulated and weakens the capacity to support a regression.

The Obsessives

Fixed anally determined attitudes defend against any expression of the components instincts, and the regressive process involved in play is inhibited. The grandiose self has been structured prematurely during the early anal period when a fantasy of the object's omnipotence is more extreme. The consequence is in a lesser degree of stability and a greater degree of susceptibility to narcissistic injury. The regression associated with symptom formation results from a breakdown in function, making play activities anxiety arousing.

The Phobias

All component instincts must be actively defended against, and the processes involved in play are either severely inhibited or unavailable. The grandiose self is prematurely structured during the oral phase, is based upon the fantasy of an all-giving nurturer, and is a highly unstable structure.

The Id (Processes of Love)

The manner in which love relationships are selected and the conditions under which they occur are the end result of an individual's developmental history. The organization of the id of the dynamic unconscious is the legacy of that history.

The Genital Character

New object-related love relationships are given depth and meaning by the representations of infantile experience that occupy the id of the dynamic unconscious. The choice of an object is no longer determined by its unconscious significance.

The Hysterias

Love objects continue to be determined by the influence of the primary attachments to infantile objects. When there is sufficient instinctual integration for symptoms to be manifested, there is some intermittent freedom from the infantile conditions of object choice. When character pathology is predominant, love relationships are inhibited due to their anxiety-arousing effect, and the choice of an object is motivated by unconscious forces.

The Obsessives

The anxiety associated with inevitable frustrations is inhibiting in all love relationships, and infantile conditions dominate the choice of an object. When obsessive symptoms have formed, love relationships are potentially traumatic and severely inhibited.

The Phobias

Love objects are determined by the search for an optimally gratifying, optimally frustrating, orally dominated infantile experience. In the object phobias, the processes of love are inhibited primarily due to the fear of rejection; in the self-phobias, it is primarily the fear of instinctual overstimulation, and in the combined self- and object phobias, it is primarily the extreme anxiety of loss of differentiation due to the regressive pull of fusion and merger.

The Superego (The Process of Work)

The ability to work is indicative of the integration of the superego and the degree of harmonious functioning with the interests of the ego. It is related to the process of selective identification and reflects the functioning of the ego ideal.

The Genital Character

Ambitions and goals operate in harmony with morals and standards in the realization of talents and skills. The ego ideal has been structured in the phallic period by including the optimally frustrating impressions of an object within self-experience, which strengthens self-regulation and gender identity. Increasingly discriminating selective identifications have successfully resolved the oedipal conflict, and the infantile representations have been replaced by the representations of new and independent objects. The superego functions as an independent regulatory and guiding agency, in full accord with the interests of the ego.

The Hysterias

Unrealized potentials are a factor in the partial work inhibitions, usually referred to as "underachieving." The ego ideal is structured late in the phallic period, when instinctual self-experiences of phallic exhibitionism become readily overstimulating. The prohibitive influences of a humiliating object are included within self-experience, and these infantile representations of an object remain firmly entrenched in the structure of the ego ideal. The super ego is polarized in its functions and acts in opposition to the interests of the ego. With the formation of symptoms, there may be some intermittent periods in which there is an integration of superego responses and ego interests, but these are generally short lasting.

The Obsessives

Anally determined reaction formations create the need to over-achieve, although the conflict engendered by assertiveness inhibits the processes involved in work. The deficiencies in sublimatory activities further accentuate that inhibition. The ego ideal, structured prematurely during the anal period, is based upon including the prohibitive influences of an anally sadistic object within self-experience. The superego remains at an early stage of organization, and its prohibitive functions are harsh and punitive. With the formation of obsessive symptoms, work is severely inhibited because there is a breakdown in the functional effectiveness of the superego.

The Phobias

The dependency upon external objects for regulation interferes with the processes involved in work, which are inordinately vulnerable to the narcissistic injuries associated with criticism and lack of recognition. The ego ideal is formed prematurely during the period of orality, is based upon the optimally gratifying impressions of a good object, functions in concert with the grandiose self, and is highly unstable. The prohibitive influences of an object are not available for regulatory functions, the superego has not consolidated into an independently functioning agency, and the infantile attachments to an object have not been replaced. The threat to cohesiveness from the influences of a bad object or from instinctual overstimulation is constantly present in the background, and work experiences are severely restricted.

Conscious Motivation for Treatment

A therapeutic situation emphasizes introspection, psychological mindedness, verbalization of internal experience, and the ability to tolerate suffering in order to gain a deeper understanding of mental events. The evolving significance of the therapeutic relationship is the primary vehicle for gaining that understanding, and interpretive communications are the therapist's primary mode of participation. The conscious motives for engaging in this endeavor are determined by and are a reflection of the underlying structural organization of the personality.

The Genital Character

There is no internal reason for this specially focused relationship and thus no conscious motivation for treatment.

The Hysterias

Psychological mindedness is present but with a diminished capacity for verbally communicating internal experience. With symptoms, there is an awareness of the internal nature of the suffering and a strong conscious motive to further the thrust of developmental progression. When hysterical character pathology is manifested, there is much anxiety associated with the process of inner exploration. The accompanying regression and increase in instinctual activity mobilize defensive responses that make the conscious motivation for treatment appear to be weak.

The Obsessives

Psychological mindedness and conceptual activity are accentuated with obsessive character pathology, although the exaggerated use of the mechanism of isolation leaves little awareness of the internal nature of the suffering. The conscious motivation to engage in a therapeutic process is weak, as an extension of anally fixed attitudes. With the regressive breakdown that results in obsessive symptoms, there is an acute awareness of the internal nature of the suffering. The need to alleviate that suffering serves as a strong conscious motive for treatment, to protect against the threat of fragmentation.

The Phobias

Conscious motivation shifts and fluctuates in accordance with the particular structural organization that is in the ascendency. In the object phobias, there is an intermittent awareness of the internal nature of the suffering, often a high degree of psychological mindedness, and a heightened sensitivity to the qualities of an interaction. Conscious motivation for treatment is strong in an empathically responsive environment and weak when empathic lapses transpire. In the self-phobias, inner exploration is associated with danger, and psychological mindedness is only intermittently present. Conscious motivation is extremely tenuous. It is strong at moments of empathic responsiveness but rapidly changes with even minimal lapses in empathy. In the combined self- and object phobias, the search for internal regulation makes self-observation difficult, and the tendency is to see suffering almost solely as a reaction to external events. Conscious motivation for treatment is weak, although there is a strong motive for sustaining a supportive relationship.

Unconscious Motivation for Treatment

This refers to the unconsciously determined motivational forces that are elicited in response to a therapeutic situation.

The Genital Character

Unconsciously determined motivating forces culminate in the selection of experiences that do not include the qualities of a therapeutic situation.

The Hysterias

The regulatory function of hysterical symptoms has facilitated a limited degree of genital instinctual integration, which is consistently interrupted by the effects of overstimulation. The unconscious motive is to enable a continuous flow of genital instinctual demand, which is expressed in the therapeutic relationship as establishing a genital instinctual attachment. The anxiety associated with this attachment mobilizes defensive responses that weaken the motivating force. With hysterical character pathology, the unconscious motive is to recreate depriving and humiliating interactions, which are designed to reinforce defensively fixed phallic attitudes. The strength of the unconscious motive is proportional to the need for reinforcement.

The Obsessives

With obsessive character pathology, the unconscious motive is to recreate sadistic interactions, which are designed to reinforce fixed anal attitudes. When there is a regressive breakdown and symptomatic compromises are formed, the unconscious motive involves the search for gratification of passive homosexual strivings. The high level of anxiety evokes defensive responses that weaken this unconscious motive.

The Phobias

The unconscious motive for treatment is fueled by the search for the influences of an orally determined good object. In an unconsciously empathic relationship, the motive is strong. Empathic lapses recreate the original trauma and abruptly weaken this unconscious motive. In the combined self- and object phobias, the need for regulation from an external object to alleviate the threatened loss of cohesiveness operates as a strong unconscious motive.

Complaints

Complaints refer to the particular manner in which a given psychic disturbance is expressed.

The Genital Character

Complaints are restricted to adaptive responses to stress, which are both transient and of short duration.

The Hysterias

The hysteric with symptoms complains of the symptoms' interference with love, work, and play. The hysteric with character pathology complains of unrealized potentials, of repetitive failures in love relationships, and of the recurrent experience of emptiness.

The Obsessives

The obsessive with character pathology complains of the demands made by significant others for greater emotional responsiveness and of periods of depression. The obsessive with symptoms complains of the fear of loss of control and of the intrusive quality of the symptoms.

The Phobias

The complaints in the phobias tend to center upon low self-esteem, emotional lability and wide mood swings, recurrent episodes of depression, and a chronic state of emptiness. There are the additional elements of the particular phobia that is predominant, which is expressed as an object phobia, claustrophobia, or a vague and ominous sense of dread. Finally, transient episodes of a loss of cohesiveness may be a factor.

This concludes the discussion of the cohesive disorders. The subtitle of this volume, *Development of Pathology in the Cohesive Disorders*, indicates that there has been sufficient structuralization within the personality for the distortions created by pathology to develop rather than emerging as a product of defect or deficiency. The influences of early development have shaped the form that these pathological distortions take but have not seriously interfered with the establishment of continuity of experience. The achievement of cohesiveness in the personality underscores the intermingling of healthy and pathological forces that are embodied in these psychic disturbances. When the destructive influences of early development are more extreme, the effect is manifested in the inability to establish cohesiveness and continuity of experience within the personality. The pathological entities that result include the borderline personality, the schizophrenias, and the autistic disorders. These expressions of pathology in the noncohesive personality will be discussed in the third volume of this series, subtitled *Pathology of Development*.

References

Abse, D. W. (1974). Hysterical conversion and dissociative syndromes and the hysterical character. In S. Ariet & E. B. Brody (Eds.), *American handbook of psychiatry* (Vol. 3, pp. 155–194). New York: Basic Books.

Arlow, J. (1963). Conflict, regression, and symptom formation. *International Journal of Psychoanalysis 44*, 12–22.

Berger, D. M. (1971). Hysteria: In search of the animus. *Comprehensive Psychiatry, 12*, 277–286.

Blocker, K. H., & Tupin, J. P. (1977). *Hysteria and hysterical structures. Developmental and social theories. Hysterical personality*. New York: Jason Aronson.

Cameron, N. (1963). *Personality development and psychopathology: A dynamic approach*. Boston: Houghton Mifflin.

Deutsch, H. (1929). The genesis of agorophobia. *International Journal of Psychoanalysis, 10*, 249–253.

Easser, B. R., & Lesser, S. R. (1965). Hysterical personality. A reevaluation. *Psychoanalytic Quarterly, 34*, 390–405.

Fenichel, O. (1945), *The psychoanalytic theory of neurosis*. New York: W. W. Norton.

Freud, A. (1965). *Normality and pathology in childhood*. New York: International Universities Press.

Freud, A. (1966). Obsessional neurosis. A summary of psychoanalytic views as presented at the congress. *International Journal of Psychoanalysis, 47*, 116–122.

Freud, A. (1977). Fears, anxieties, and phobic phenomena. *Psychoanalytic study of the child* (Vol. 32). New York: International Universities Press.

Freud, S. (1953). A case of hysteria. Three essays on sexuality. In J. Strachey (Ed. and Trans.), *The standard edition of the complete psychological works of Sigmund Freud* (Vol. 7). London: Hogarth Press. (Original work published 1901–1905)

Freud, S. (1955). Three contributions to the theory of sex. In J. Strachey (Ed. and Trans.), *The standard edition of the complete psychological works of Sigmund Freud* (Vol. 2). London: Hogarth Press. (Original work published 1910)

Freud, S. (1959). The predisposition of obsessional neurosis. In J. Strachey (Ed. and Trans.), *The standard edition of the complete psychological works of Sigmund Freud* (Vol. 9). London: Hogarth Press. (Original work published 1924)

Freud, S. (1963). Character and anal eroticism. In J. Strachey (Ed. and Trans.), *The standard edition of the complete psychological works of Sigmund Freud* (Vol. 15). London: Hogarth Press. (Original work published 1915)

Greenson, R. (1959). Phobias, anxiety, and depression. *Journal of the American Psychoanalytic Association, 7,* 663–674.

Grotstein, J. (1981). *Splitting and projective identification.* New York: Jason Aronson.

Horowitz, M. (1977). *Hysterical personality.* New York: Jason Aronson.

Jones, E. (1913). *Papers on psychoanalysis* (1st ed.). New York: Wood and Co.

Kernberg, O. (1970). Factors in the psychoanalytic treatment of narcissistic personalities. *Journal of the American Psychoanalytic Association, 18,* 51–85.

Kernberg, O. (1976). *Object relations theory and clinical psychoanalysis.* New York: Jason Aronson.

Kohut, H. (1971). *The analysis of the self.* New York: International Universities Press.

Lazare, A. (1971). The hysterical character in psychoanalytic theory. Evolution and confusion. *Archives of General Psychiatry, 25,* 131–137.

Marmor, J. (1953). Orality in the hysterical personality. *Journal of the American Psychoanalytic Association, 1,* 656–675.

Nagera, H. (1981). *The developmental approach to childhood psychopathology.* New York: Jason Aronson.

Rangell, L. (1959). The nature of conversion. *Journal of the American Psychoanalytic Association. 17,* 632–662.

Reich, W. (1933). *Character analysis.* New York: Farrar, Strauss, and Giroux.

Rothstein, A. (1979). Oedipal conflicts in narcissistic personality disorders. *International Journal of Psychoanalysis, 60,* 189–199.

Sandler, J., & Joffe, M. B. (1965). Notes on obsessional manifestations in children. *Psychoanalytic study of the child* (Vol. 20, pp. 425–438). New York: International Universities Press.

Sperling, M. (1973). Conversion hysteria and conversion symptoms. A revision and classification and concepts. *Journal of the American Psychoanalytic Association, 21,* 745–772.

Wangh, M. (1967). Psychoanalytic thought on phobia: Its evolution and its relevance for therapy. *American Journal of Psychiatry, 123* (9), 1075–1080.

Zetzel, E. (1968). The so-called good hysteric. *International Journal of Psychoanalysis, 49,* 256–260.

Index